Medical Management
of Glaucoma

Medical Management of Glaucoma

Keith Barton
Consultant Ophthalmologist
Moorfields Eye Hospital Foundation Trust
Honorary Reader
Department of Epidemiology and Genetics
Institute of Ophthalmology
University College London
London, UK

Roger A Hitchings
Past President, European Glaucoma Society
Emeritus Professor of Glaucoma and Allied Studies
University College London
Honorary Consultant Ophthalmologist
Moorfields Eye Hospital
London, UK

Editor
Donald L Budenz
Kittner Distinguished Professor and Chair of Ophthalmology
UNC Health Care System
Chapel Hill, NC, USA

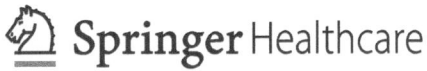 Springer Healthcare

Published by Springer Healthcare Ltd, 236 Gray's Inn Road, London, WC1X 8HB, UK.

www.springerhealthcare.com

© 2013 Springer Healthcare, a part of Springer Science+Business Media.

British Library Cataloguing-in-Publication Data.

A catalogue record for this book is available from the British Library.

ISBN 978-1-858734-30-9

Although every effort has been made to ensure that drug doses and other information are presented accurately in this publication, the ultimate responsibility rests with the prescribing physician. Neither the publisher nor the authors can be held responsible for errors or for any consequences arising from the use of the information contained herein. Any product mentioned in this publication should be used in accordance with the prescribing information prepared by the manufacturers. No claims or endorsements are made for any drug or compound at present under clinical investigation.

Project editor: Tess Salazar
Designer: Joe Harvey
Artworker: Sissan Mollerfors
Production: Marina Maher
Printed in Great Britain by Latimer Trend

Contents

Author biographies   vii

Abbreviations   ix

Foreword   x

1 Introduction   **1**

Definition of glaucoma   1

The scale of the problem   4

Quality of life for patients with glaucoma   6

Factors contributing to late diagnosis of glaucoma   8

Classification of glaucoma   11

An overview of the classes of glaucoma   15

Risk factors for glaucoma   25

References   29

2 Pathogenesis of glaucoma   **33**

Determinants of intraocular pressure   33

Aqueous humor production and outflow in the healthy eye   34

Disturbances in aqueous humor production and outflow   38

Variations in intraocular pressure   44

Ocular blood flow and glaucoma   46

References   48

3 Diagnosing glaucoma   **49**

History   49

Overview of assessments used in the diagnosis of glaucoma   50

Pachymetry   51

Slit-lamp examination   52

Tonometry   53

Gonioscopy   56

Dilated fundus examination and optic disc evaluation   60

Automated perimetry   67

Investigating ocular perfusion   67

Conclusions 69

References 69

4 Medical management of glaucoma 71

Overview 71

Principles of medical management of glaucoma 74

Current therapeutic options for glaucoma 85

Improving adherence in patients with glaucoma 91

Cost of glaucoma therapy 95

Management of emergency situations 95

Mechanisms to improve quality of life during treatment of glaucoma 96

Follow-up 96

References 99

Author biographies

Keith Barton, MD is a Consultant Ophthalmologist at the Moorfields Eye Hospital, and is an Honorary Reader for the Department of Epidemiology at the Institute of Ophthalmology, University College London. Additionally, Dr Barton is the Chairman of the International Glaucoma Association, a registered charity for people with glaucoma.

Keith Barton is a Glaucoma Specialist whose research interests include the surgical management of glaucoma, specifically secondary glaucoma and the use of aqueous shunt devices, and the management of cataract in glaucoma.

Roger A Hitchings, MD is an Honorary Consultant Ophthalmologist at Moorfields Eye Hospital, London and Professor Emeritus in Glaucoma and Allied studies at the University of London. He was Director of Research and Development at Moorfields Eye Hospital.

As a glaucoma specialist, he has a special interest in optic nerve imaging, visual field progression, glaucoma surgery, and normal tension glaucoma. He has also carried out research into the effect of topically applied medications on the conjunctiva and the success of glaucoma surgery. He has authored and edited 4 books, including the *Atlas of Clinical Ophthalmology* (with Dr David J Spalton and Dr Paul Hunter; winner of "BMA Medical Book of the Year", 2005) and the two volume book *Glaucoma* (coeditors Dr Tarek Shaarawy, Dr Mark B Sherwood, and Dr Jonathan G Crowston), 15 book chapters, and over 200 peer-reviewed papers on glaucoma.

Roger Hitchings developed the glaucoma department at Moorfields Eye Hospital into the largest in the UK and one of the largest in the world. It now functions with ophthalmologists and scientists, representing all aspects of subspecialization in glaucoma.

He is currently past president of the European Glaucoma Society, and Founder Member of the World Glaucoma Association (AIGS).

As Director of Research and Development, he had responsibility for establishing the Clinical Trials Unit and the associated Reading Centre. The latter has become one of the key centers for the evaluation of ophthalmic clinical trials in the UK. He was responsible for developing the Royal College of Ophthalmologists' 5 year Strategic Plan for Eye research, which set out research goals in the specialty.

He has delivered a number of invited lectures, including:

- 1997 "Duke Elder Lecture" Annual Meeting Royal College of Ophthalmologists
- 2000 Shaffer Lecture American Academy of Ophthalmology Annual meeting
- 2001 Guest Lecturer honoring George L Spaeth at the American Glaucoma Society
- 2002 Ida Mann Lecture Oxford
- 2006 Goldmann Lecture Glaucoma Research Society Vancouver
- 2008 Bowman Lecture Royal College of Ophthalmologists
- 2009 Bartisch Lecture University of Dresden

Donald L Budenz, MD, MPH is the Kittner Distinguished Professor and Chair of the Department of Ophthalmology, University of North Carolina in Chapel Hill. Dr Budenz completed medical school at Harvard and was trained in ophthalmology at the University of Pennsylvania's Scheie Eye Institute. He performed a glaucoma fellowship at the Bascom Palmer Eye Institute, University of Miami School of Medicine where he subsequently became Professor of Ophthalmology and Associate Medical Director. He completed a Master in Public Health at the Johns Hopkins Bloomberg School of Public Health. Dr Budenz has authored over 130 peer reviewed scientific articles, numerous book chapters, and a single-authored textbook entitled *Atlas of Visual Fields*. His areas of research include medical testing for glaucoma, epidemiology of eye disease, and clinical trials in glaucoma surgery.

Abbreviations

AAO	American Academy of Ophthalmology
APAC	Acute primary angle-closure
AGIS	Advanced Glaucoma Intervention Study
CAI	Carbonic anhydrase inhibitors
CCT	Central corneal thickness
CPAC	Chronic angle-closure or chronic primary angle-closure
CPACG	Chronic primary angle-closure glaucoma
DOPP	Diastolic ocular perfusion pressure
GAT	Goldmann applanation tonometry
GON	Glaucomatous optic neuropathy
IOP	Intraocular pressure
MAOI	Monoamine oxidase inhibitors
NPG	Normal-pressure glaucoma
NTG	Normal-tension glaucoma
OHT	Ocular hypertension
ORA	Ocular response analyzer
PACG	Primary angle-closure glaucoma
PGA	Prostaglandin analogue
POAG	Primary open-angle glaucoma
RGC	Retinal ganglion cells
SWAP	Short wavelength automated perimetry
WHO	World Health Organization

Foreword

This single volume textbook provides a short introduction to the ophthalmic subspecialty area: glaucoma. It does not claim to be comprehensive, but sets out to give the ophthalmology resident and other healthcare professionals a guide to the subject. It is to be hoped that it will stimulate the reader to look at original sources of information in specific areas within the subspecialty, and, hopefully generate interest for the them to develop specialist expertise of their own.

Chapter 1

Introduction

Definition of glaucoma

The term glaucoma encompasses a number of diseases in which there is a progressive loss of retinal ganglion cells (RGC) with corresponding visual field loss that results in a characteristic "cupped" appearance in the optic nerve head. Glaucoma results in an irreversible loss of visual field, usually starting in the periphery (Figure 1.1) [1], and sometimes affecting the central visual field first (Figure 1.2), but leading to varying degrees of visual disability and, in a small but significant proportion of patients, blindness.

This damage to the optic nerve is often but not always associated with an increase in intraocular pressure (IOP). In the past, the term glaucoma was often confined to patients with IOP elevation; however, generally this is no longer the case because it is recognized that the role played by IOP varies from patient to patient. Some optic nerves appear to withstand sustained mild IOP elevation for many years without obvious damage, whereas others will develop optic neuropathy when the IOP has never been outside the normal range (known as normal-tension or normal-pressure glaucoma [NTG or NPG]; see page 17). There appears to be no difference in the morphometric appearance between eyes that have glaucoma in association with elevated IOP and those with NTG. These two syndromes are now believed to represent one disease spectrum, and lowering IOP in eyes with NTG has proven to be beneficial in preventing progression.

K. Barton and R. A. Hitchings, *Medical Management of Glaucoma*,
DOI: 10.1007/978-1-907673-44-3_1, © Springer Healthcare 2013

The visual field in glaucoma

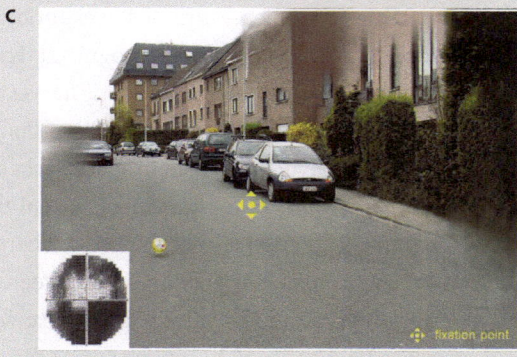

Figure 1.1 The visual field in glaucoma. Visual field examinations and corresponding images showing the likely effect on visual function in a normal eye (**A**), and an eye affected by an early (**B**), or later stage of glaucoma (**C**). The yellow symbols in B and C represent the patient's fixation point. Objects located completely in the blind areas are not seen. These areas are filled-in with the colors and patterns of the surrounding area. Reproduced with permission from © Ann Hoste, 2013 [1]. All Rights Reserved.

Paracentral visual field defects in glaucoma

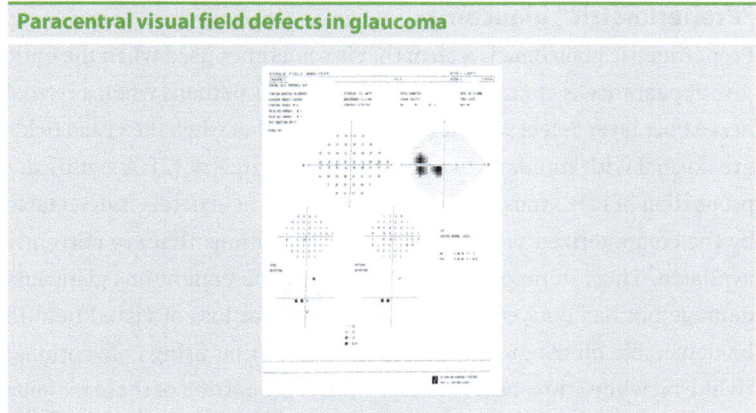

Figure 1.2 Paracentral visual field defects in glaucoma. Enlargement of the blind spot may be an early sign of glaucoma, as seen in this visual field example; however, of much greater significance is the early paracentral visual field defect. Progression of this defect may lead to functional visual loss much earlier than the stereotypical peripheral visual field defects that are illustrated in Figure 1.1. Reproduced with permission from © Moorfields Eye Hospital, 2013. All Rights Reserved.

Patients who have glaucomatous damage but normal IOP levels tend to be diagnosed later in the course of the disease; this is likely due to the fact that since IOP elevation is absent, the examiner is not alerted to the possibility of glaucoma during a routine refraction examination (see page 8–10). Such late presentation has led to the development of the term "sneak thief of sight" due to the slow, painless and relentless nature of the condition that may not manifest until vision is severely impaired.

The only proven method of preventing progression of glaucoma, at the time of writing, is the reduction of IOP, whether by medical or surgical means. In the majority of glaucoma cases, lowering the IOP is expected to reduce the likelihood of further damage and thereby stabilize the condition. It is uncertain, at present, if there is a level below which further reduction of IOP is ineffective, although there is some evidence that patients with glaucoma progress relatively rarely when the IOP level is consistently in the low normal range.

This book will review the classification (Chapter 1), pathogenesis (Chapter 2), diagnosis (Chapter 3) and management of primary open-angle glaucoma (POAG) (Chapter 4) in the context of medical management of IOP levels.

"Preperimetric" glaucoma

Preperimetric glaucoma is a term that is sometimes used when the optic disc appearance is characteristic of glaucoma or perhaps when a retinal nerve fiber layer defect is visible on fundoscopy, but when the visual fields are normal with standard "white on white" perimetry [2]. A significant proportion of RGCs must be lost before a visual field defect is detectable by the computerized visual field-testing algorithms that are currently available. Thus, in preperimetric glaucoma, the patient has glaucoma damage but has not yet lost sufficient RGCs for loss of visual field to be detectable on computerized visual field testing using conventional "white on white" threshold perimetry [3]. A proportion of these patients will demonstrate visual field loss using other modalities, such as short wavelength automated perimetry (SWAP), a modality that uses a blue stimulus on a yellow background; however, defects detected using SWAP are less specific for the diagnosis of glaucoma than those detected with "white on white" perimetry. Therefore, SWAP is only used in clinical practice in combination with other tests, and in this way false-positive SWAP diagnoses can be avoided.

Although visible structural changes in the optic disc are often manifest before changes in the visual field become apparent, this is not always the case. In addition, there is a significant overlap in the appearance of the optic nerve head between normal and abnormal. Thus, in the early stages of glaucoma, both structural and functional measurements are often required to make the diagnosis with certainty.

The scale of the problem

According to the World Health Organization (WHO), glaucoma is the second leading cause of blindness worldwide when refractive error is excluded, behind cataracts; glaucoma was also the leading cause of irreversible blindness, ahead of macular degeneration [4,5]. The contribution of glaucoma to the incidence of worldwide blindness is illustrated in Figure 1.3 [5,6].

In one European population-based study, the 5-year risk of developing open-angle glaucoma was measured at 1% in those aged 60 years but rose to approximately 3% for those aged 80 years [7]. In those with

Global causes of blindness as a proportion of total blindness in 2002

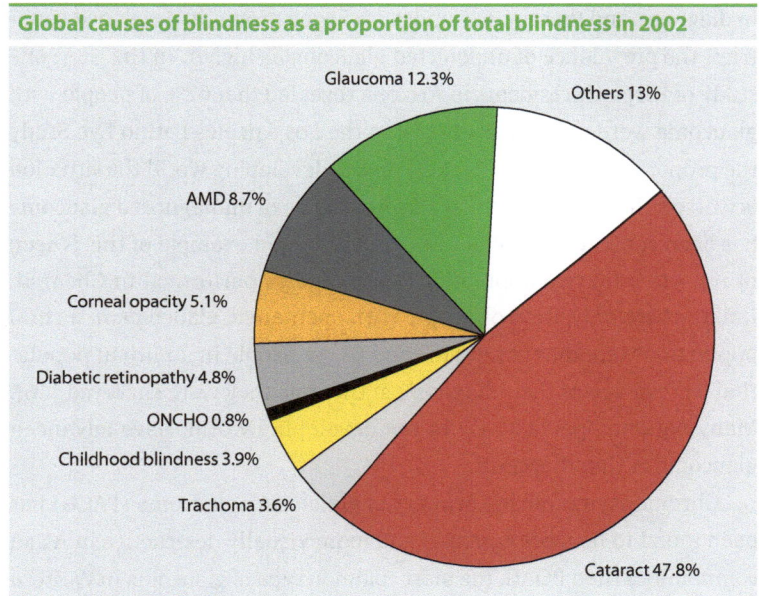

Figure 1.3 Global causes of blindness as a proportion of total blindness in 2002.
AMD, age-related macular degeneration; ONCHO, Onchocerciasis. Reproduced with permission from © World Health Organization, Resnikoff et al, 2013 [5]. All Rights Reserved.

an affected eye, the 5-year risk of developing glaucoma in the other eye is five times higher than for unaffected individuals. Approximately 480,000 individuals aged 40 years and older are estimated to have glaucoma in England and Wales alone [8]. Population-based studies suggest an overall prevalence of open angle glaucoma in the US population of 40 years and older of 1.86%, with 398,000 blacks and 1.57 million whites affected [6]. In 2006, Quigley and Broman calculated that by 2010 there would be roughly 60 million sufferers of glaucoma worldwide, increasing to 80 million by 2020, with individuals of Sub-Saharan African descent being disproportionately affected [9].

The prevalence of undetected glaucoma is very high. Approximately half of all glaucoma sufferers in the developed world are unaware of their condition, a figure that has proved remarkably consistent in epidemiological studies (50% in the Melbourne visual impairment project [10]; 51% in the Blue Mountains Eye Study [11]; and 53% in the Rotterdam Eye Study [12]); there is no evidence that this has improved despite improvements in diagnosis and therapy. For underprivileged groups in developed countries, the prevalence of undetected glaucoma is higher. In the USA, one study of Hispanic residents in Arizona revealed that 62% of people with glaucoma were undiagnosed [13]; in the Los Angeles Latino Eye Study the proportion was over 75% [14]. In the developing world the situation is worse still to the extent that the prevalence of undiagnosed glaucoma has been consistently greater than 80%. A good example of this is seen in reports from two population-based studies performed in Chennai, India, where only 1.5% of people with open-angle glaucoma in a rural population were diagnosed [15] and 6% of people in an urban population were aware of their diagnosis at the time they were surveyed [16]. Many patients, particularly in the developing world, have advanced glaucoma at first diagnosis.

Chronic asymptomatic primary angle-closure glaucoma (PACG) has been found to be more common and more visually destructive in Asian communities than POAG, the most common type of glaucoma in Western societies, or even symptomatic PACG [17,18].

The economic burden of glaucoma is substantial. It has been calculated at US$2.9 billion in direct medical costs in the US alone in one year (2004) [19]; the economic costs of glaucoma rises to just over US$6 billion when nonmedical costs and loss of productivity are taken into account as well. In the UK, it has been calculated that over £300 million was spent on the management of glaucoma in 2002: 45% of costs were associated with direct medical costs, 20% with direct nonmedical costs, and 35% with indirect costs [20]. In the EU and the USA costs have been related to stage of the disease. In developing countries costs are held down by 1) inability to pay, 2) generic drugs, 3) the early surgery option, 4) underdiagnosis. While generic drugs have only recently begun to dominate EU and US markets, some larger developing countries have traditionally had a thriving generic market.

Quality of life for patients with glaucoma

The impact of glaucoma on quality of life is considerable and is often underestimated (as summarized in Table 1.1) [21–28]. Even patients with mild visual field defects have been shown to demonstrate reduced mobility [29]; however, provided that the visual field is not significantly restricted by the time of diagnosis, patients with glaucoma can lead a normal life. In most patients it is possible to slow glaucomatous progression significantly, if not halt it completely, with treatment. In order to achieve this, the patient must adhere to long-term treatment regimens and must be regularly monitored, which have an impact on quality of life (Table 1.1) [1,21–28]. If left untreated, glaucoma can have a devastating

Quality of life issues in patients with glaucoma	
Issues related to diagnosis	
Patient perceptions and overall quality of life	• Patients with glaucoma report decreased quality of life [21–26]. Some of this is due to visual field loss [26]; however, the impact of the diagnosis can adversely affect quality of life. A Japanese study reported that elderly patients' quality of life was reduced due to loss of hopes for future life and consequences of the disease more so than just the symptoms of the disease alone [24]
Decreased functional ability, mobility and loss of independence [22]	• Bilateral glaucoma is associated with falls, slower walking, bumping into objects and, in some studies, with higher accident rates [27] (eg, one study showed 2.4 m/minute slower walking speed through an obstacle course and 1.65 times the number of bumps compared with persons without glaucoma [$P<0.05$ for both] [28])
	• Drivers with glaucoma are significantly more likely to change their driving habits with regard to driving at night, on motorways and in unfamiliar areas [1]
	• In some countries (eg, the UK), patients with bilateral glaucoma must inform driver licensing authorities and may have to undergo tests to assess whether vision is sufficient to continue driving
Issues related to treatment - the daily need for medication and the impact of surgery may also affect quality of life	
Inconvenience of treatment	• Disruption to normal day-to-day life by time-consuming eye drop administration patterns, frequent appointments and lengthy tests
Side effects	• Stinging, blurring, redness and soreness of the eyes are not uncommon with eye drops. Surgery may reduce vision for a period after the procedure
Cost	• In some countries where treatment costs are not completely met by state/insurance providers, cost considerations may reduce adherence

Table 1.1 Quality of life issues in patients with glaucoma. Adapted from Hoste [1], Altangerel et al [21], Nutheti et al [22], Gupta et al [23], Uenishi et al [24], McKean-Cowdin et al [25], Freeman et al [26], Ramulu [27], and Friedman et al [28].

effect on quality of life because it can eventually lead to blindness. For example, the WHO estimated glaucoma to be responsible for 18% of blindness both in Europe and the United States, in 2002, based on available epidemiological data [5]. In the United States, glaucoma is estimated to be responsible for 6.4% of all cases of blindness in whites, 26% of cases in African Americans and 28.6% of cases in Hispanics [30].

Factors contributing to late diagnosis of glaucoma

The natural consequence of a high prevalence of undiagnosed glaucoma, as mentioned above, is late presentation; unfortunately, many cases of glaucoma are diagnosed late in the disease process, by which time serious visual field loss has occurred and central vision is threatened.

There are a number of reasons for late diagnosis (Table 1.2) [31,32]. The major one is absence of symptoms in the early stages.

Absence of symptoms

Glaucoma in its early stages is usually asymptomatic. Many individuals with glaucoma may have symptoms related to other common ocular conditions, such as presbyopia, posterior vitreous detachments or blepharitis, but glaucoma may remain asymptomatic until large areas of the visual field are lost. One exception to this is the patient with early paracentral visual defects close to fixation (Figure 1.2), who may notice symptoms of a positive scotoma early in the course of disease. Such a patient is generally at a higher risk of central vision loss and will need more aggressive treatment. However, normal visual acuity does not preclude the presence

Reasons for late diagnosis of glaucoma
1. Lack of symptoms in early-to-mid stages: • peripheral vision affected first so central vision is preserved until late stages; • both eyes are not affected equally; and • cerebrocortical plasticity
2. Poor sensitivity of screening tests
3. Diminishing vision is often accepted as a consequence of aging
4. Irregular eye examinations
5. Occupational status
6. Lack of family history of glaucoma

Table 1.2 Reasons for late diagnosis of glaucoma. Adapted from Fraser et al [31,32].

of glaucoma, and visual field loss can be severe even in patients who have normal Snellen visual acuity.

Absence of symptoms may also be due to the asymmetrical nature of the disease in that advanced glaucoma may be missed in one eye if the fellow eye has good vision. This asymmetry may result in failure to notice relatively advanced glaucoma in one eye because of good vision in the fellow eye.

In congenital field defects or those acquired early in life, it has long been believed that cortical plasticity allows the brain to *fill in* the missing gaps in the field so they are not noticed [33]. There is now some evidence that this also happens with acquired defects. In essence, the brain "papers over the cracks" to complete the picture so that no defect is noticed. This is well-illustrated in Figure 1.4 and is responsible for the failure of the patient with glaucoma represented in Figure 1.1 to see the child, yet he or she is are unaware of the loss of that part of the

Demonstration of cortical plasticity

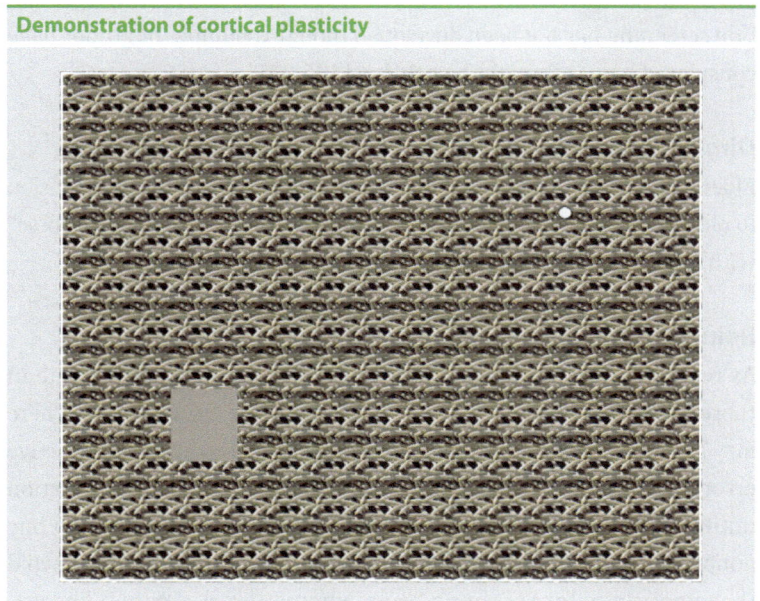

Figure 1.4 Demonstration of cortical plasticity. With strict fixation at the white fixation point the homogenous gray square vanishes within 10 seconds and gets replaced by the pattern from the surrounding background. Reproduced with permission from © Ann Hoste, 2013 [1]. All Rights Reserved.

visual field [1]. For that reason, patients with advanced glaucoma may have relatively marked visual field defects without being aware of them.

Sensitivity and specificity of screening tests

While in developed countries, much glaucoma is detected by so-called opportunistic screening (eg, during routine optometric examination), to date there is no cost-effective strategy of population screening for glaucoma [34]. There is no IOP level that provides a reasonable balance of sensitivity and specificity for detecting glaucoma [35] and many cases would be missed if case-detection were attempted using IOP alone. Individual structural and functional tests do not have sufficiently high sensitivity and specificity to identify early glaucoma. The diagnosis is a clinical judgment, based on the collective evidence from a number of test results, including quantitative measurement of visual field defects and IOP, and the visible appearance of the retina and optic nerve head on slit lamp examination (see Chapter 3). To date, cost effective population screening has not been developed though a number of groups have considered how this might be achieved [36,37].

Diminishing vision often associated with increasing age

Elderly individuals with glaucoma may attribute their diminishing vision to old age. It is often assumed by the public that the eyes will get "worse" with age, and so the elderly do not always seek assistance.

Reluctance to have regular eye tests

As reported by Fraser, glaucoma is most likely to be diagnosed late in those individuals who do not have regular routine eye tests [31]. There may be a number of reasons for this; however, subjects with no refractive error (ie, emmetropic individuals) are unlikely to attend for refraction until they become presbyopic, and even then, the recent trend to buy nonprescription reading glasses may permit such individuals to avoid the opportunity for screening by an optometrist or ophthalmologist. Fraser et al attempted to identify risk factors for late presentation, using case-control methodology [31,32,38]. They reported a linear trend of increasing odds of late presentation associated with increasing Standard

Occupational Classification [31]. Those presenting late were less likely to be in managerial and skilled occupations than unskilled. They were also less likely to have a family history of glaucoma than those presenting early, and were less likely to have visited an optometrist. Overall, both late diagnosis and glaucoma blindness are inextricably associated with lower income, though there are additional reasons for late diagnosis as outlined above.

Classification of glaucoma

Glaucomas are usually classified as:

- **primary or secondary,** according to whether there is an identifiable underlying ocular or systemic disorder causing the glaucoma (secondary) or not (primary);
- **open-angle or closed-angle (angle closure),** according to the mechanism of IOP elevation (ie, whether there is a clinically visible anatomical obstruction to aqueous outflow in the iridocorneal drainage angle [angle closure] or not [open-angle]) (Table 1.3) [39]; and
- **developmental (congenital),** the developmental glaucomas are often considered as a separate group, each with specific causes and therapeutic approaches.

Glaucomas can also be classified by severity. Angle-closure glaucoma can be further classified according to the mechanism of closure (Table 1.3) [2].

In the European Union and the United States, POAG is by far the most common type of glaucoma; exfoliation syndrome (pseudoexfoliation), pigment dispersion, uveitis and iris neovascularization are important secondary causes. In contrast, primary angle-closure is more prevalent than open-angle glaucoma in Asia [9].

Classification as primary or secondary glaucoma

Primary glaucoma usually affects both eyes, though often asymmetrically, and is often but not always associated with IOP elevation. In contrast, secondary glaucomas are due to IOP elevation as a result of aqueous outflow obstruction caused by another ocular or systemic disorder. The

Classification of glaucoma based on mechanisms of outflow obstruction

Open-angle glaucoma mechanisms

Pretrabecular (membrane overgrowth)	Trabecular	Posttrabecular

• Fibrovascular membrane (neovascular glaucoma)	• Idiopathic
	  – Chronic open-angle glaucoma
	  – Juvenile open-angle glaucoma
		• Obstruction of Schlemm's canal (eg, collapse at canal)

• Endothelia layer, often with Descemet-like membrane
  – Iridocorneal endothelial syndrome
  – Posterior polymorphous dystrophy
  – Penetrating and nonpenetrating trauma
	• "Clogging" of trabecular meshwork
	  – Red blood cells
	    – Hemorrhagic glaucoma
	    – Ghost cell glaucoma
	    – Sickle red blood cells
	  – Macrophages
	    – Hemolytic glaucoma
	    – Phacolytic glaucoma
	    – Melanomalytic glaucoma
	  – Neoplastic cells
	    – Primary ocular tumors
	    – Neoplastic tumors
	    – Juvenile xanthogranuloma
		• Elevated episcleral venous pressure
		  – Carotid cavernous fistula
		  – Cavernous sinus thrombosis
		  – Retrobulbar tumors
		  – Thyroid ophthalmopathy
		  – Superior vena cava obstruction
		  – Mediastinal tumors
		  – Sturge-Weber syndrome
		  – Familial episcleral venous pressure elevation

• Epithelial downgrowth	– Pigment particles
	    – Pigmentary glaucoma
	    – Exfoliation syndrome (glaucoma capsulare)
	    – Malignant melanoma	

• Fibrous ingrowth	– Protein
	    – Uveitis
	    – Lens-induced glaucoma	

• Inflammatory membrane
  – Fuchs heterochronic iridocyclitis
  – Luetic interstitial keratitis
	– Viscoelastic agents alpha-Chymotrypsin–induced glaucoma	

	• Alterations of the trabecular meshwork
	  – Steroid-induced glaucoma
	  – Edema
	    – Uveitis (trabeculitis)
	    – Scleritis and episcleritis
	    – Alkali burns	

	• Trauma (angle recession)	
	• Intraocular foreign bodies (hemosiderosis, chalcosis)	

Table 1.3 Classification of glaucoma based on mechanisms of outflow obstruction. Clinical examples cited in this table do not represent an inclusive list of the glaucomas. This article was published in *The Glaucomas*, Second edition, Ritch et al, © Elsevier (1996) [2].

Angle-closure glaucoma mechanisms

Anterior ("pulling")	Posterior ("pushing")	Developmental anomalies of anterior chamber angle

• Contracture of membranes
  – Neovascular glaucoma
  – Iridocorneal endothelial syndrome
  – Posterior polymorphous dystrophy
  – Penetrating and nonpenetrating trauma
• Consolidation of inflammatory products
	• With pupillary block
	  – Pupillary-block glaucoma
	  – Lens-induced mechanisms
	    – Phacomorphic lens
	    – Ectopia lentis
	  – Posterior synechia
	    – Iris–vitreous block
	    – Pseudophakia
	    – Uveitis
	• Without pupillary block
	  – Ciliary block (malignant) glaucoma
	  – Lens-induced mechanisms
	    – Phacomorphic lens
	    – Ectopia lentis
	  – Following lens extraction (forward vitreous shift)
	  – Anterior rotation of ciliary body
	    – Following sclera buckling
	    – Following panretinal photocoagulation
	    – Central retinal vein occlusion
	  – Intraocular tumors
	    – Malignant melanoma
	    – Retinoblastoma
	  – Cysts of the iris and ciliary body
	  – Retrolenticular tissue contracture
	    – Retinopathy of prematurity (retrolental fibroplasia)
	    – Persistent hyperplastic primary vitreous
		• Incomplete development of trabecular meshwork–Schlemm's canal
		  – Congenital (infantile) glaucoma
		  – Axenfeld-Rieger syndrome
		  – Peters anomaly
		  – Glaucomas associated with other developmental anomalies
		• Iridocorneal adhesions
		  – Broad strands (Axenfeld-Rieger syndrome)
		  – Fine strands that contract to close angle (aniridia)

IOP elevation in secondary glaucoma is commonly asymmetrical, often unilateral and may lead to much more rapid visual loss than POAG [39].

Primary angle-closure and secondary causes of IOP elevation should be distinguished from primary glaucomas because secondary glaucomas are often treated differently. Thus, in secondary glaucoma, treatment is directed both toward the primary disease as well as the glaucoma. In primary angle-closure, treatment is primarily directed at breaking the angle closure episode [39].

The major types of primary and secondary glaucoma are reviewed later in this chapter.

Classification by severity

As glaucoma is a chronic, progressive disease affecting only one organ, clinical staging is always somewhat arbitrary. Many classification systems have been devised for staging severity and field loss (for a detailed review, see Brusini and Johnson [40]) [11]. While no single system is in widespread use, it is helpful to have a working method of classifying severity because it is important to identify patients who have more severe visual loss at presentation as they have a higher risk of progression of visual loss.

In general, those with advanced glaucoma require more aggressive treatment than those with less advanced glaucoma, and surgical management is generally considered much earlier in these patients.

The simplest classifications use mean deviation on standard automated perimetry. This gives an overall impression of the state of the visual field; however, this type of classification would categorize patients as mild if they had a small visual field defect close to fixation, whereas such patients are actually at a high risk of visual loss. A number of classifications have attempted to base severity on both the degree of visual field loss and the location of the loss.

The Hodapp, Parrish and Anderson classification [41] is a more sophisticated method, based on two criteria. The first is the overall extent of the damage (calculated by using mean deviation and the Humprey-Statpac-2 pattern deviation probability map). The second is based on the proximity of the visual field defect to the point of fixation. Another widely-quoted system is the Advanced Glaucoma Intervention Study (AGIS) classification system [42]. These types of classification systems are generally used for research rather than clinical practice. The clinician often classifies the patient in practice according to the overall extent of visual field loss (eg, using mean deviation) and whether or not fixation is threatened. An example of a system for classifying the severity of glaucoma is given in Table 1.4.

While it is widely agreed that a defect close to fixation represents a serious risk and should thereby be classified in the advanced category, the levels of mean deviation used are somewhat arbitrary.

An overview of the classes of glaucoma

Primary glaucoma

Primary glaucoma may occur in eyes with open or closed iridocorneal angles. In POAG there is no visible obstruction to the outflow of aqueous humor on gonioscopy. The reduction in outflow is caused by reduced function in the trabecular meshwork outflow pathway. In primary angle-closure, the iridocorneal angle is obstructed by the peripheral iris,

Glaucoma severity	
Type of glaucoma	**Definition**
Early glaucoma	• Visible structural optic disc damage, either optic disc cupping. In some eyes with small optic discs, retinal nerve fiber layer loss may be seen in the absence of visible disc cupping • Normal or mildly abnormal field on (MD > –5 dB) on standard automated perimetry
Moderate glaucoma	• Visible structural optic disc damage and associated retinal nerve fiber layer loss • Moderate peripheral visual field loss on standard automated perimetry. No defect close to fixation (MD –5 to –10 dB)
Advanced glaucoma	• Marked structural optic disc damage. Extensive visual field loss or any visual field defect close to central fixation • Loss of central vision loss is not necessary for glaucoma to be categorized as "advanced" (MD < –10 dB)

Table 1.4 Glaucoma severity. This table gives a rough definition of the characteristics of early, moderate and advanced (severe) glaucoma; there are a number of classification systems, and staging is a clinical judgment based on evaluation of all the available clinical data. Mean deviation is the mean reduction in threshold sensitivity on visual field testing with standard automatic perimetry as compared to a normal population. dB, decibels; MD, mean deviation.

preventing aqueous humor from accessing the trabecular meshwork and exiting the eye. Because these two broad classes of glaucoma are managed differently, gonioscopy is essential when assessing all patients with glaucoma at the initial visit and periodically throughout the course of the disease. The pathological processes involved in these two classes of glaucoma are described in more detail in Chapter 2.

Primary open-angle glaucoma

POAG, formerly known as chronic simple or chronic open-angle glaucoma, is the most common type of glaucoma, accounting for approximately 75% of cases worldwide [9]. The disease usually develops slowly over years with gradual RGC and visual field loss. There is no cure; treatment aims to slow progression but cannot reverse existing damage [43].

Peripheral (outer) field loss often occurs first (see Figure 1.1), with central vision usually affected relatively late in the course of the disease; however, as discussed previously in this chapter, this is not always the case. Some patients develop paracentral visual field defects in advance of significant peripheral loss, and consequently have a higher risk of loss of central vision. Hence, any patient with a visual field defect close to fixation at diagnosis is immediately categorized as having "advanced glaucoma".

POAG usually occurs in both eyes, but the extent of disease is often greater in one eye than the other. Many patients present with significant vision loss at diagnosis. The relative risk of POAG rises exponentially with rises in IOP, and there is no evidence of a specific threshold IOP for the onset of the condition [44]. For a discussion of normal and abnormal IOP levels see Chapter 2.

There are a number of clinical presentations of POAG. These vary from patients with suspicious optic discs and normal IOP to those with elevated IOP and normal optic discs and to those with glaucomatous optic neuropathy (GON) with or without elevated IOP:

- POAG with elevated IOP (normal IOP being ≤21 mmHg);
- POAG with normal IOP (NTG or NPG);
- ocular hypertension (OHT); and
- POAG suspect.

This classification is somewhat arbitrary. Patients with OHT may never develop glaucoma, but are included in this list of presentations because elevated IOP is *the* major risk factor for POAG. Each of the classes is described below.

Primary open-angle glaucoma with elevated intraocular pressure

POAG, with or without elevated IOP, is characterized by a slow loss of RGCs, resulting in visual field loss, and also a characteristic appearance of cupping of the optic disc. While the average rate of field loss is related to the average degree of IOP elevation, individual patients vary greatly in the rate of progression. Men and women are affected equally. Untreated POAG may lead eventually to blindness.

Primary open-angle glaucoma with normal intraocular pressure (normal-tension or normal-pressure glaucoma)

Many would now dispute that NTG and NPG are separate entities; however, the term has persisted in clinical use partly because it is sometimes helpful to remember when treating these patients that a lower than usual target IOP level may be required if a high untreated IOP has never been documented. By definition, risk factors other than IOP must exist in patients with NTG, where GON develops at IOP levels that are statistically in the normal range, albeit often toward the upper end of the normal range.

As one might expect, in eyes of patients with low levels of IOP, progression is usually slow, but may be detected in 10% of cases within a follow-up period as short as 1 year [44]. No detectable progression is observed within 5 years in approximately 30% of patients [44]; however, severe visual impairment may occur. When IOP measurement has been the sole method of case detection, these patients have often been diagnosed late.

Ocular hypertension

By definition, patients with OHT have had documented IOP levels greater than the normal range on at least one and sometimes more occasions without evidence of GON. The terminology and guidelines of the European Glaucoma Society [45] recommend that the term OHT should be restricted to IOP that is consistently greater than two to three standard deviations above the population mean *when all other ocular findings are within normal limits* (within the normal range, for example, optic disc and cup size). The higher the IOP, the greater the risk is of developing POAG. The important point here is "population mean"; this differs between the Japanese or West African where it is lower to Europeans where it is higher. In the United States, OHT is diagnosed when the IOP is consistently two standard deviations above the population mean, or greater than 21 mmHg.

Primary open-angle glaucoma suspect

As a result of better examination and imaging techniques and increased awareness, many subjects presenting to the clinician with possible glaucoma are labeled as POAG suspects. These are usually patients with normal visual fields and normal or borderline IOP levels whose optic disc appearance is abnormal in appearance. In some patients the cup:disc ratio is larger than normal, and this often occurs in the presence of a larger than average optic nerve head (>2.0 mm vertical diameter). Another common scenario is the patient with myopia and a stretched or tilted optic disc in which the cup is not centered in the disc and one or more segments of the rim are thinner than usual [46,47]. The difficulty in differentiating POAG suspect from someone with definite POAG is therefore the presence of an abnormal optic disc in the absence of other features of glaucoma.

Usually, in such patients the retinal nerve fiber layer and visual field will both be normal; however, in some circumstances patients with tilted myopic discs may also have associated visual field defects, either because of the anomalous disc architecture or from associated myopic chorioretinal degeneration, which further confuse the situation. In these patients, only sequential examination and analysis over time can differentiate those with progressive glaucoma from those who have a stationary optic disc abnormality.

Primary angle-closure glaucoma

The main subject of this book, chronic POAG, is the most common type of glaucoma in Europe and the United States, and thus a detailed discussion of PACG is beyond the scope of the book; however, its classification and pathogenesis are briefly described here and in Chapter 2, respectively.

There are three broad clinical courses that PACG may follow:

- acute primary angle-closure (APAC);
- intermittent primary angle-closure; and
- chronic primary angle-closure (CPAC).

Acute primary angle-closure

APAC usually presents with a dramatic rise in IOP, often accompanied by iris ischemia and inflammation. Although the condition presents acutely, the patient usually gives symptoms of worsening headache, nausea, vomiting, visual disturbances, severe eye pain and red eyes over a course of several days (Figure 1.5).

Development of APAC is a medical emergency; it is difficult to reverse effectively and immediate medical attention is required as there is high risk of severe permanent damage to the affected eye. The treatment options in the acute stage involve medical therapy with topical aqueous suppressants, alpha-agonists, parasympathomimetics and systemic carbonic anhydrase inhibitors, and hyper-osmotic agents. Laser or surgical iridotomy is almost always required. Laser iridoplasty, anterior chamber paracentesis and trabeculectomy are other procedures that are often used to break the attack.

Acute primary angle-closure

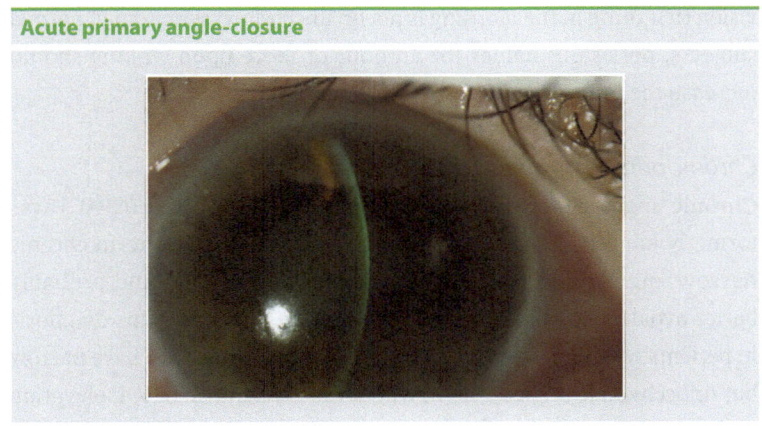

Figure 1.5 Acute primary angle-closure. Reproduced with permission from © Michael Compton, MD, 2013. All Rights Reserved.

In cases of pupillary block (see below and Chapter 2), iridotomy should be sufficient to prevent recurrence of the pupil block; however, the IOP may remain elevated if significant peripheral anterior synechia have developed during the period of iridotrabecular apposition. Angle closure secondary to plateau iris, although managed similarly in the acute phase, often recurs due to forward rotation of the ciliary processes. While many cases also involve a degree of pupillary block, iridotomy may not be sufficient to prevent recurrence and often iridoplasty, cataract surgery or filtration surgery and/or chronic topical pilocarpine, are required to prevent recurrence of angle closure.

Intermittent primary angle-closure

This is also known as subacute angle-closure and is often more difficult to diagnose and, therefore, is easily missed. This is because the IOP is often normal during the eye examination. This type of angle closure may present with optic disc cupping in the presence of a normal IOP and the diagnosis is only made after a careful history and gonioscopy with a high index of suspicion.

The principal symptoms are headache and blurring of vision or haloes in the vision upon waking or occasionally late at night, as intermittent angle closure tends to occur at night when the pupil dilates in dim light and the chance of iridotrabecular contact is greatest. While blurring of vision first thing in the morning is not an uncommon symptom in normal subjects, persistent haloes for an hour or more upon waking should increase the index of suspicion.

Chronic primary angle-closure

Chronic angle-closure or chronic primary angle-closure (CPAC) was formerly known as chronic narrow angle glaucoma. The term chronic narrow angle glaucoma is imprecise, less often used, and probably better avoided because of a common practice of making this diagnosis in patients with POAG who coincidentally were observed to have narrow but unoccludable angles, and in whom the mechanism of IOP elevation is clearly different from those with true CPAC.

Otherwise, CPAC is symptomatically similar to POAG (Figure 1.6). Chronic and permanent damage evolves from CPAC into chronic primary angle-closure glaucoma (CPACG)

Developmental glaucoma

The term developmental glaucoma usually refers to primary glaucomas arising in childhood or infancy, although they occasionally occur in young adulthood (secondary glaucomas of childhood are as diverse as those of adults [48]). For primary developmental glaucomas, the

Chronic primary angle-closure

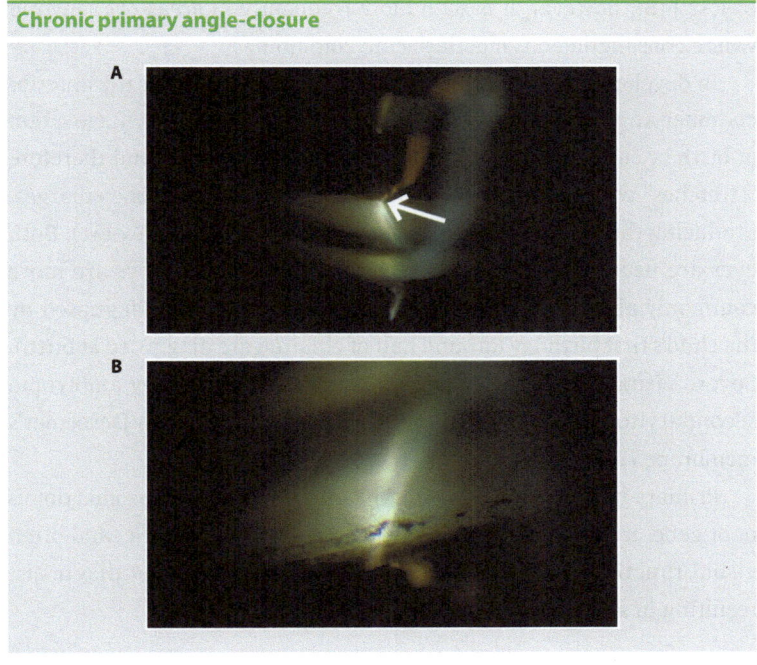

Figure 1.6 Chronic primary angle-closure. Photographs showing the gonioscopic appearance in two quadrants of an eye with chronic primary angle-closure. As is often the case in this condition, the entire circumference of the angle is not completely closed. **A,** while the upper angle is completely closed, as seen the apex of the corneoscleral transition zone marks the position of Schwalbe's line and in this photograph (arrow) coincides with the position where the iris meets the angle, indicating that the angle is closed in this area; **B,** shows the lower part of the angle in the same eye. This angle is open in the area illustrated, but pigmentation of the angle indicates that there is also likely to be intermittent iridotrabecular contact. Reproduced with permission from © Moorfields Eye Hospital, 2013. All Rights Reserved.

classification used in the current European Glaucoma Society terminology and guidelines [45] is:

- *Primary congenital glaucoma* – presenting at birth or up to the age of 9 years;
- *Primary juvenile glaucoma* – presenting between 10 and 35 years of age.

In the literature, the term infantile glaucoma is also used for primary congenital glaucoma developing during childhood.

Primary congenital glaucoma is relatively rare, with an estimated prevalence in the United States of 1.46 per 100,000 people aged 20 years or less [48]; however, it is seen more frequently in areas of the world where consanguineous marriages are common.

In developmental glaucoma, abnormal development of the anterior chamber angle results in reduced aqueous outflow and IOP elevation at birth or early childhood. The growing sclera is elastic and therefore "stretches" with IOP elevation, with the result that the globe enlarges, producing the characteristic appearance of buphthalmos (*ox-eye*). Both eyes are usually, but often asymmetrically, involved. Boys are more commonly affected than girls. This condition is usually diagnosed by the child's first birthday (around half of children are diagnosed at birth). Severe visual disability is common, and often caused by amblyopia secondary to central corneal opacification from splits in Descemet's membrane (Haab's striae) and refractive errors.

Primary juvenile glaucoma may be inherited as an autosomal dominant gene. It is associated with myopia but is asymptomatic, and often visual function has been irreversibly lost by the time of diagnosis, resulting in significant disability.

Secondary glaucomas

Secondary glaucomas develop as a result of other ocular conditions, trauma or intraocular surgery, or as a complication of a systemic disease (eg, diabetes mellitus) or a side effect of medical treatment (eg, corticosteroids). Diagnosis and management of the secondary glaucomas is outside the scope of this book; however, examples of some of the more significant secondary glaucomas are summarized in Table 1.5 and Figure 1.7.

Summary of significant types of secondary glaucoma

Type of glaucoma	Characteristics
Secondary open-angle	
Exfoliation (pseudoexfoliation) syndrome	• Fibrillar material is deposited throughout the eye, including the trabecular meshwork, and is most easily visible on the anterior lens surface after pupil dilation. Iris pigment is also abraded from the pupil margin and deposited on the anterior iris surface and trabecular meshwork • IOP is often higher than in POAG • Prevalence increases with age
Pigment dispersion syndrome and pigmentary glaucoma	• Iris pigment is abraded from the posterior surface of the peripheral iris by the zonules during accommodation. The abraded pigment deposits on various surfaces within the eye, including the trabecular meshwork • IOP elevation may never develop. The risk of developing IOP elevation has been found to be up to 37% • More common in men than women, usually young myopes
Glaucoma due to trauma	• For example, blunt, nonpenetrating trauma to the eye may result in tearing of the anterior ciliary body (angle recession) • Eyes with angle recession have an elevated risk of glaucoma that may develop many years after the original trauma
Corticosteroid-induced glaucoma	• Long-term use of topical or systemic corticosteroids can elevate IOP as a consequence of increased resistance to aqueous outflow. IOP usually returns to normal after discontinuation of the drug. The length of time taken for the IOP to normalize may be prolonged if the patient has been using corticosteroids for a prolonged period
Glaucoma secondary to elevated episcleral venous pressure	• Secondary IOP elevation can rarely occur as a result of obstruction of venous drainage of the eye, such as a carotid-cavernous sinus fistula or other arteriovenous anomaly
Secondary angle-closure glaucoma	
Neovascular glaucoma	• Iris and angle neovascularization usually occur as a complication of either diabetes or retinal vein occlusion • Less common causes are retinal vasculitis and ocular ischemic syndrome • Neovascular glaucoma is often particularly aggressive and difficult to treat
Glaucoma secondary to uveitis	• Glaucoma is a common complication of uveitis. The mechanism may be open or closed • Acute-angle closure secondary to pupillary block is an especially devastating complication of uveitis (see Figure 1.7)
Iridocorneal endothelial syndrome	• Abnormal corneal endothelium causes unilateral glaucoma with iris atrophy and corneal edema • Patients are young to middle-aged

Table 1.5 Summary of significant types of secondary glaucoma. IOP, intraocular pressure; POAG, primary open-angle glaucoma.

Acute angle closure secondary to complete pupillary block in a case of uveitis with a secluded pupil

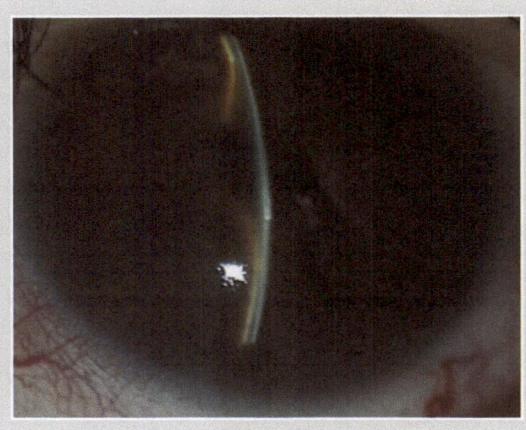

Figure 1.7 **Acute angle closure secondary to complete pupillary block in a case of uveitis with a secluded pupil.** Reproduced with permission from © Moorfields Eye Hospital, 2013. All Rights Reserved.

Mixed-mechanism glaucoma

In a proportion of patients, glaucoma may result from a number of mechanisms. Uveitic glaucoma is an especially good example as the patient may develop IOP elevation from any combination of a number of causes. Open-angle mechanisms include swelling of the trabecular meshwork beams, corticosteroid treatment, clogging of the trabecular meshwork by inflammatory cells, or damage to the trabecular meshwork from inflammation. Angle closure may occur acutely from pupillary block or chronically from synechial development or sometimes angle occlusion by an inflammatory or neovascular membrane.

Complicated cataract surgery is another good example where IOP elevation might develop. This may be due to a combination of aphakia, uveitis, retained lens cortex or nucleus, angle closure, or iris pigment abrasion by a sulcus-fixated lens haptic.

In primary glaucoma, the mechanism is also sometimes uncertain; a patient with a narrow or closed angle that has been successfully treated without residual synechia may have persistent IOP elevation afterward if an episode of high IOP during an angle closure episode has been sufficient to damage the trabecular meshwork to the extent that its function is permanently reduced, even when the angle is open. Although it is also possible for a patient to have open-angle glaucoma in the presence of narrow angles, it is important to exclude intermittent-angle closure as a cause of IOP elevation in these patients.

Risk factors for glaucoma

A number of risk factors for glaucoma have been identified by population-based studies. These are listed in Table 1.6 [6,9,49–57].

Intraocular pressure elevation

Most cases of glaucoma are associated with elevated IOP; however, a proportion of individuals develop glaucomatous optic nerve damage with no documented evidence of IOP elevation. Overall, in prevalence studies, NTG accounts for 20–39% of individuals with glaucoma (Figure 1.8) [58]. While NTG or NPG is no longer considered a separate entity from POAG, rather part of the POAG disease spectrum, it is sometimes helpful

Risk factors for glaucoma	
Risk factor	**Notes**
Modifiable	
IOP elevation	• IOP elevated in most but not all glaucomatous eyes
Systemic hypertension and other vascular factors	• A risk factor for glaucoma, but one whose role has not yet been fully elucidated
Unmodifiable	
Age	• IOP rises in most people >40 years • Increasing glaucoma risk with increasing age
Ethnic origin	• Elevated IOP more common with African origin • African, East Asian and Hispanic patients are at higher glaucoma risk than Caucasians
Family history of glaucoma	• Raised glaucoma risk if parental or sibling has elevated IOP levels
Myopia	• Raised glaucoma risk with moderate-to-high myopia
CSF pressure	• Low CSF pressure may have an effect on axoplasmic transport that is similar to that of elevated IOP

Table 1.6 Risk factors for glaucoma. CSF, cerebrospinal fluid; IOP, intraocular pressure. Adapted from Friedman et al [6], Quigley and Broman [9], Mitchell et al [49], Mitchell [50], Flammer et al [51], Leske et al [52], Leske et al [53], Wilson et al [54], Wormald et al [55], Doshi et al [56], and Berdahl et al [57].

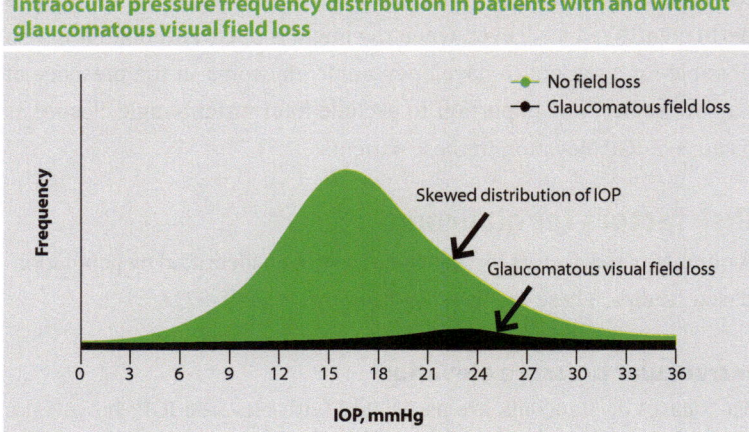

Figure 1.8 Intraocular pressure frequency distribution in patients with and without glaucomatous visual field loss. The *black area* represents patients who have glaucomatous visual field loss, and the *green area* represents patients without glaucomatous visual field loss. Note that a very low percentage of individuals with normal pressure (IOP ≤21 mmHg) have field loss; however, only about 10% of patients with elevated pressure have field loss. It is evident that the proportion of the population with field loss is greater in higher-pressure ranges. For example, the proportion is approximately 30% at 30 mmHg but increases to 50% at 35 mmHg. Note that the average pressure among those with glaucoma is approximately 23 mmHg, and about one third of patients with glaucoma have pressures within the normal range. IOP, intraocular pressure. Adapted from Gedde et al [58].

when evaluating the effects of treatment that these patients have normal untreated IOP levels and often lower treatment target IOP levels are set [46].

The relationship between IOP levels and glaucoma is discussed in more detail in Chapter 2; tonometry to measure IOP is described in Chapter 3; and approaches to the management of glaucoma by reducing IOP are discussed in Chapter 4.

Systemic hypertension and other vascular factors

It is accepted that the only modifiable risk factor for primary glaucomas is the degree of IOP elevation; however, the Australian Blue Mountains Eye Study found a doubling of the 10-year incidence of glaucoma in the eyes of patients with uncontrolled systemic hypertension as compared to those with controlled blood pressure [49,50]. An analysis of over 27,000 patients in a practice database noted that hypertension was more likely to be found in those who later developed glaucoma (odds ratio, 1.29) [51].

Vascular dysregulation has been proposed to be a primary cause of reduced ocular blood flow in glaucoma [51]. Circulatory problems appear to be more common in patients with glaucomatous damage than in age-matched controls. This is especially true of patients with NTG; however, the exact role of vascular factors in the pathogenesis is uncertain.

There is some evidence that low ocular perfusion pressure is a positive predictive factor for the development of visual field loss in defined populations (see Chapter 2) [52,53]. It is possible that poor ocular perfusion may increase the susceptibility of the optic nerve to damage; however, there is no evidence to support treatment of glaucoma by manipulating perfusion pressure [45,59].

Nonmodifiable risk factors

Age

Increasing age is the most important single risk factor for glaucoma. The development and progression of glaucomatous damage is highly age-dependent because the cumulative loss of retinal ganglion fibers during a lifetime increases with age.

The prevalence is between four and ten times higher in the oldest age groups compared with younger age groups [60]. For example, in the Beaver Dam Eye Study of a white population in the USA, the prevalence increased from 0.9% in people of 43–54 years old to 4.7% in those 75 years of age or older [61]. In the Baltimore Eye Survey, a US population-based prevalence survey of other 5000 individuals over 40 years of age, the prevalence increased from 0.92% in 40- to 49-year olds to 2.16% in those aged 80 years or older; in the same study, the rates for the black population were 1.23% and 11.26%, respectively [62].

At the time of writing, many developed countries face a huge increase in the demand for glaucoma service provision because of changing demographics with an aging population.

Ethnic origin

Individuals of African origin are more likely to have elevated IOP than other ethnic groups [55]. The Baltimore Eye Survey found that the prevalence of glaucoma was 4–5 times higher in blacks than whites. The prevalence was 11% in blacks aged 80 years or more. Glaucoma appears to occur earlier in people of African origin than in whites [62]. Individuals of East Asian or Hispanic origin are also at a higher risk than whites, and Asians account for approximately half of all glaucoma sufferers [9].

NTG is relatively common in populations of European origin [61]. Certain forms of glaucoma are more prevalent in different racial or ethnic groups:

- NTG seems to be much more common in Japanese people than in Europeans;
- PACG is more common in East Asian and Chinese populations; and
- pigmentary glaucoma is more common in light-skinned individuals than in dark-skinned individuals.

Gender
There is a slight gender predilection for certain types of glaucoma. For example, pigmentary glaucoma is more common in men, whereas primary angle-closure is slightly more common in women. Most population-based prevalence studies have found a higher prevalence of POAG in women [6] that disappears after age-adjustment. One study even found a reversal of this apparent predilection when corrected for the longer life-expectancy of women (age-adjusted male:female ratio of 1.4 in the Barbados Eye Study [63]). Overall, there appears to be no predilection for POAG toward either gender [6].

Family history of glaucoma and genetic predisposition
First-degree relatives of glaucoma patients have a higher risk than individuals without a family history; however, studies vary greatly in their estimates of the association with family history, partly because of patients' recall bias and also because relatives of glaucoma sufferers are more likely to present for ophthalmic examination than individuals with no family history.

The most accurate estimates come from population-based studies. In the Baltimore Eye Study, the odds ratio of developing open-angle glaucoma was 3.69 for those with affected siblings and 2.17 for those with affected parents [63].

Genetic mutations associated with primary glaucomas include MYOC, OPTN and WDR36. More recently mutations and single nucleotide polymorphisms in the LMX1B transcription factor gene have been reported to be associated with POAG. Dominant mutations in the latter also cause Nail-Patella syndrome.

Myopia and hypermetropia

Myopia has proven an inconsistent risk factor for glaucoma in epidemiological studies. Presently, low myopia does not appear to be a significant risk factor, whereas moderate-to-high myopia (>3–4 diopters) is associated with an increased risk of POAG. Myopia is also a risk factor for pigmentary glaucoma.

Hyperopia carries an increased risk of PACG. Hyperopic eyes are also at a higher risk of developing aqueous misdirection (malignant glaucoma) after intraocular surgery.

Cerebrospinal fluid pressure

Recent evidence suggests that the pressure gradient between the vitreous cavity and meninges may also influence optic nerve function. As the optic nerve is bathed in CSF, CSF pressure is thought to provide a degree of resistance to posterior bowing of the lamina cribrosa in response to high IOP (ie, CSF pressure provides a supporting function when the lamina cribrosa is being pushed posteriorly by high IOP). It may also be that low CSF pressure when the IOP is normal, may have a similar effect to elevating the IOP levels, even in the absence of changes in ocular blood perfusion pressure [57]. This hypothesis could explain optic disc cupping in the presence of normal IOP.

References

1   Hoste AM. New insights into the subjective perception of visual field defects. *Bull Soc Belge Ophthalmol.* 2003;287:65-71.

2   American Academy of Ophthalmology: The Eye M.D. Association. In: *2008-2009 Basic and Clinical Science Course, Section 10: Glaucoma.* San Francisco, CA: American Academy of Ophthalmology; 2011.

3   Kerrigan-Baumrind LA, Quigley HA, Pease ME, et al. Number of ganglion cells in glaucoma eyes compared with threshold visual field tests in the same persons. *Invest Ophthalmol Vis Sci.* 2000;41:741-748.

4   World Health Organization. Magnitude and causes of visual impairment. Fact Sheet N°282. 2011. Available at www.who.int/mediacentre/factsheets/fs282/en/. Accessed August 7, 2013.

5 Resnikoff S, Pascolini D, Etya'ale D, et al. Global data on visual impairment in the year 2002. *Bull World Health Organ.* 2004;82:844-851.

6 Friedman DS, Wolfs RC, O'Colmain BJ, et al. Prevalence of open-angle glaucoma among adults in the United States. *Arch Ophthalmol.* 2004;122:532-538.

7 de Voogd S, Ikram MK, Wolfs RCW, et al. Incidence of open-angle glaucoma in a general elderly population: the Rotterdam Study. *Ophthalmology.* 2005;112:1487-1493.

8 National Collaborating Centre for Acute Care. NHS. National Institute for Health and Clinical Excellence. Glaucoma: Diagnosis and management of chronic open angle glaucoma and ocular hypertension. Available at: www.nice.org.uk/nicemedia/pdf/CG85NICEGuideline.pdf. Published April 2009. Accessed August 7, 2013.

9 Quigley HA, Broman AT. The number of people with glaucoma worldwide in 2010 and 2020. *Br J Ophthalmol.* 2006;90:262-267.

10 Wensor MD, McCarty CA, Stanislavsky YL, et al. The prevalence of glaucoma in the Melbourne Visual Impairment Project. *Ophthalmology.* 1998;105:733-739.

11 Mitchell P, Smith W, Attebo K, et al. Prevalence of open-angle glaucoma in Australia. The Blue Mountains Eye Study. *Ophthalmology.* 1996; 103:1661-1669.

12 Dielemans I, Vingerling JR, Wolfs RC, et al. The prevalence of primary open-angle glaucoma in a population-based study in The Netherlands. The Rotterdam Study. *Ophthalmology.* 1994;101:1851-1855.

13 Quigley HA, West SK, Rodriguez J, et al. The prevalence of glaucoma in a population-based study of Hispanic subjects: Proyecto VER. *Arch Ophthalmol.* 2001;119:1819-1826.

14 Varma R, Ying-Lai M, Francis BA, et al. Prevalence of open-angle glaucoma and ocular hypertension in Latinos: the Los Angeles Latino Eye Study. *Ophthalmology.* 2004;111:1439-1448.

15 Vijaya L, George R, Paul PG, et al. Prevalence of open-angle glaucoma in a rural south Indian population. *Invest Ophthalmol Vis Sci.* 2005;46:4461-4467.

16 Vijaya L, George R, Baskaran M, et al. Prevalence of primary open-angle glaucoma in an urban south Indian population and comparison with a rural population. The Chennai Glaucoma Study. *Ophthalmology.* 2008;115:648-654.

17 Thomas R, Sekhar GC, Parikh R. Primary angle-closure glaucoma: a developing world perspective. *Clin Exp Ophthalmol.* 2007;35:374-378.

18 Foster PJ, Baasanhu J, Alsbirk PH, et al. Glaucoma in Mongolia. A population-based survey in Hovsgol province, northern Mongolia. *Arch Ophthalmol.* 1996;114:1235-1241.

19 Rein DB, Zhang P, Wirth KE, et al. The economic burden of major adult visual disorders in the United States. *Arch Ophthalmol.* 2006;124:1754-1760.

20 Rouland JF, Berdeaux G, Lafuma A. The economic burden of glaucoma and ocular hypertension: implications for patient management: a review. *Drugs Aging.* 2005;22:315-321.

21 Altangerel U, Spaeth GL, Rhee DJ. Visual function, disability, and psychological impact of glaucoma. *Curr Opin Ophthalmol.* 2003;14:100-105.

22 Nutheti R, Shamanna BR, Nirmalan PK, et al. Impact of impaired vision and eye disease on quality of life in Andhra Pradesh. *Invest Ophthalmol Vis Sci.* 2006;47:4742-4748.

23 Gupta V, Srinivasan G, Mei SS, et al. Utility values among glaucoma patients: an impact on the quality of life. *Br J Ophthalmol.* 2005;89:1241-1244.

24 Uenishi Y, Tsumura H, Miki T, et al. Quality of life of elderly Japanese patients with glaucoma. *Int J Nurs Pract.* 2003;9:18-25.

25 McKean-Cowdin R, Wang Y, Wu J, et al. Los Angeles Latino Eye Study Group. Impact of visual field loss on health-related quality of life in glaucoma: the Los Angeles Latino Eye Study. *Ophthalmology.* 2008;115:941-948.

26 Freeman EE, Muñoz B, West SK, et al. Glaucoma and quality of life. The Salisbury Eye Evaluation. *Ophthalmology.* 2008;115:233-238.

27 Ramulu P. Glaucoma and disability: which tasks are affected, and at what stage of disease? *Curr Opin Ophthalmol.* 2009;20:92-98.

28 Friedman DS, Freeman E, Munoz B, et al. Glaucoma and mobility performance: the Salisbury Eye Evaluation Project. *Ophthalmology*. 2007;114:2232-2237.

29 Noe G, Ferraro J, Lamoureux E, et al. Associations between glaucomatous visual field loss and participation in activities of daily living. *Clin Experiment Ophthalmol*. 2003;31:482-486.

30 The Eye Diseases Prevalence Research Group. Causes and prevalence of visual impairment among adults in the United States. *Arch Ophthalmol*. 2004;122:477-485.

31 Fraser S, Bunce C, Wormald R. Risk factors for late presentation in chronic glaucoma. *Invest Ophthalmol Vis Sci*. 1999;40:2251-2257.

32 Fraser S, Bunce C, Wormald R. Retrospective analysis of risk factors for late presentation of chronic glaucoma. *Br J Ophthalmol*. 1999;83:24-28.

33 Ramachandran VS, Gregory RL. Perceptual filling in of artificially induced scotomas in human vision. *Nature*. 1991;350:699-702.

34 Healey PR. Screening for Glaucoma. In: Shaarawy T, Sherwood MB, Hitchings RA, Crowston JG, eds. *Glaucoma*. New York, NY: Elsevier; 2009:15-23.

35 Burr JM, Mowatt G, Hernández R, et al. The clinical effectiveness and cost-effectiveness of screening for open angle glaucoma: a systematic review and economic evaluation. *Health Technol Assess*. 2007;11:iii-iv, ix-x, 1-190.

36 Tielsch JM, Katz J, Singh K, et al. A population-based evaluation of glaucoma screening: the Baltimore Eye Survey. *Am J Epidemiol*. 1991;134:1102-1110.

37 The Glaucoma Screening Platform Study Group. Developing the clinical components of a complex intervention for a glaucoma screening trial: a mixed methods study. *BMC Med Res Methodol*. 2011;11:54.

38 Vaahtoranta-Lehtonen H, Tuulonen A, Aronen P, et al. Cost effectiveness and cost utility of an organized screening programme for glaucoma. *Acta Ophthalmol Scand*. 2007;85:508-518.

39 Fraser S, Bunce C, Wormald R, Brunner E. Deprivation and late presentation of glaucoma: case-control study. *BMJ*. 2001;322:639-643.

40 Brusini P, Johnson CA. Staging functional damage in glaucoma: review of different classification methods. *Surv Ophthalmol*. 2007;52:156-179.

41 Hodapp E, Parrish RK, Anderson DR. *Clinical decisions in glaucoma*. St Louis, MO: The C.V. Mosby Co.; 1993:52-61.

42 The AGIS Investigators. Advanced glaucoma intervention study. 2. Field scoring and reliability. *Ophthalmology*. 1994;101:1445-1455.

43 Weinreb RN, Khaw PT. Primary open-angle glaucoma. *Lancet*. 2004;363:1711-1720.

44 Hitchings RA. A practical approach to the management of normal tension glaucoma. In: Grehn F, Stamper R, eds. *Essentials in Ophthalmology: Glaucoma*. Berlin, Germany: Springer-Verlag; 2004.

45 European Glaucoma Society. *Terminology and Guidelines for Glaucoma*. 3rd edition. Savona, Italy: Dogma; 2008.

46 Quigley HA, Enger C, Katz J, et al. Risk factors for the development of glaucomatous visual field loss in ocular hypertension. *Arch Ophthalmol*. 1994;112:644-649.

47 Jonas JB, Bergua A, Schmitz-Valckenberg P, et al. Ranking of optic disc variables for detection of glaucomatous optic nerve damage. *Invest Ophthalmol Vis Sci*. 2000;41:1764-1773.

48 Brandt JD. Congenital glaucoma. In: Yanoff M, Duker JS, eds. *Ophthalmology*. London, UK: Mosby; 1999.

49 Mitchell P, Lee AJ, Rochtchina E, et al. Open-angle glaucoma and systemic hypertension: the Blue Mountains Eye Study. *J Glaucoma*. 2004;13:319-326.

50 Mitchell P. Session 2. The infinite improbability drive – Epidemiology Co-Chairs: Richard Wormald and Paul Chew. Diabetes, blood pressure caffeine: Is it or is it not! The Glaucoma Galaxy: A Hitch-Hikers Guide – Perspectives from a career under pressure. In: Barton K, ed. *International Glaucoma Review: The Journal for the World Glaucoma Association*. 2008;10-1:20-22.

51 Flammer J, Haefliger IO, Orgül S, Resink T. Vascular dysregulation: a principal risk factor for glaucomatous damage? *J Glaucoma*. 1999;8:212-219.

52 Leske MC, Heijl A, Hyman L, et al. EMGT Group. Predictors of long-term progression in the early manifest glaucoma trial. *Ophthalmology*. 2007;114:1965-1972.

53 Leske MC, Wu SY, Nemesure B, et al. Incident open-angle glaucoma and blood pressure. *Arch Ophthalmol.* 2002;120:954-959.

54 Wilson MR, Gallardo M. Glaucoma risk factors: ethnicity and glaucoma. In: Schacknow PN, Samples JR, eds. *The Glaucoma Book: A Practical Evidence-Based Approach to Patient Care.* New York, NY: Springer Science+Business Media, LLC; 2010:101-109.

55 Wormald RP, Basauri E, Wright LA, et al. The African Caribbean Eye Survey: risk factors for glaucoma in a sample of African Caribbean people living in London. *Eye.* 1994;8:315-320.

56 Doshi V, Ying-Lai M, Azen SP, et al; the Los Angeles Latino Eye Study Group. Sociodemographic, family history, and lifestyle risk factors for open-angle glaucoma and ocular hypertension: the Los Angeles Latino Eye Study. *Ophthalmology.* 2008;115:639-647.

57 Berdahl JP, Allingham RR, Johnson DH. Cerebrospinal fluid pressure is decreased in primary open-angle glaucoma. *Ophthalmology.* 2008;115:763-768.

58 Gedde SJ, Budenz DL, Anderson DR. Primary open-angle glaucoma and normal-tension glaucoma. In: Parrish R II, Budenz DL, eds. *The University of Miami Bascom Palmer Eye Institute Atlas of Ophthalmology.* Philadelphia, PA: Current Medicine Group LLC; 2000.

59 Caprioli J, Coleman AL; Blood Flow in Glaucoma Discussion. Blood pressure, perfusion pressure, and glaucoma. *Am J Ophthalmol.* 2010;149:704-712.

60 Fraser S, Wormald R. Epidemiology of glaucoma. In Yanoff M, Duker JS, eds. *Ophthalmology.* London, UK: Mosby; 1999.

61 Klein BE, Klein R, Sponsel WE, et al. Prevalence of glaucoma. The Beaver Dam Eye Study. *Ophthalmology.* 1992;99:1499-1504.

62 Tielsch JM, Sommer A, Katz J, et al. Racial variations in the prevalence of primary open-angle glaucoma. The Baltimore Eye Survey. *JAMA.* 1991;266:369-374.

63 Leske MC, Connell AM, Schachat AP, et al. The Barbados Eye Study. Prevalence of open angle glaucoma. *Arch Ophthalmol.* 1994;112:821-829.

Chapter 2

Pathogenesis of glaucoma

The factors that determine the development of retinal/optic nerve damage and loss of visual function have not been fully identified. While the intraocular pressure (IOP) level is the major risk factor, other issues such as the tolerance of retinal ganglion cells (RGCs) in the individual patient, the role of the supporting connective tissue at the lamina cribrosa, autoregulation of local blood supply, and perfusion pressure are likely to play a part. This chapter reviews IOP as the major factor in the pathogenesis of glaucoma with a brief overview of ocular blood flow and perfusion pressure.

Determinants of intraocular pressure

As discussed in Chapter 1, glaucoma is usually, although not invariably, associated with IOP elevation. Three factors that determine IOP are:
1. the rate of aqueous humor production by the ciliary body;
2. resistance to aqueous humor outflow across the trabecular meshwork-Schlemm's canal system (the juxtacanalicular meshwork is generally thought to be the site of greatest resistance); and
3. the level of episcleral venous pressure.

IOP elevation is generally due to increased aqueous outflow resistance, as discussed below.

K. Barton and R. A. Hitchings, *Medical Management of Glaucoma*, DOI: 10.1007/978-1-907673-44-3_2, © Springer Healthcare 2013

Aqueous humor production and outflow in the healthy eye

Aqueous humor production

Aqueous humor is produced by the ciliary body and fills the anterior chamber (the space between the cornea and the iris) and posterior chamber (the space between the iris and lens) (Figures 2.1, 2.2) [1].

Each of the approximately 80 ciliary processes comprises a double layer of epithelium (the outer layer is pigmented, the inner layer is not) over a core of stroma and a rich supply of fenestrated capillaries. These capillaries are supplied mainly by branches of the major arterial circle of the iris [1]. The apical surfaces of the outer and inner layers of the epithelium are joined by tight junctions, which are a fundamental part of the blood–aqueous barrier [1]. The inner epithelial layer protrudes into the posterior chamber and comprises of cells containing numerous mitochondria and microvilli; these cells are thought to be the site of aqueous humor production [1].

The formation of aqueous humor and its secretion across the large surface area of the ciliary processes into the posterior chamber occurs as a result of active secretion, ultrafiltration and simple diffusion. Active secretion requires energy (hydrolysis of adenosine triphosphate) to

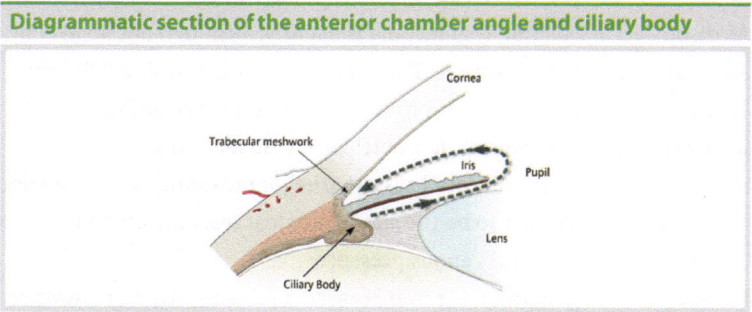

Diagrammatic section of the anterior chamber angle and ciliary body

Figure 2.1 Diagrammatic section of the anterior chamber angle and ciliary body. Dotted line shows the normal path of aqueous humor, which is actively produced in the epithelium of the ciliary body, passes through the posterior chamber between lens and iris, into the anterior chamber to exit the eye passively via the trabecular meshwork to Schlemm's canal and into the venous system. A small proportion of aqueous in the human eye also exits through the root of the iris and the ciliary muscle, into the suprachoroidal space (uveoscleral outflow). Courtesy of Alan Lacey, reproduced with permission from © Moorfields Eye Hospital, 2013. All Rights Reserved.

Cross section of the anterior segment of the normal eye, showing sites of normal aqueous outflow

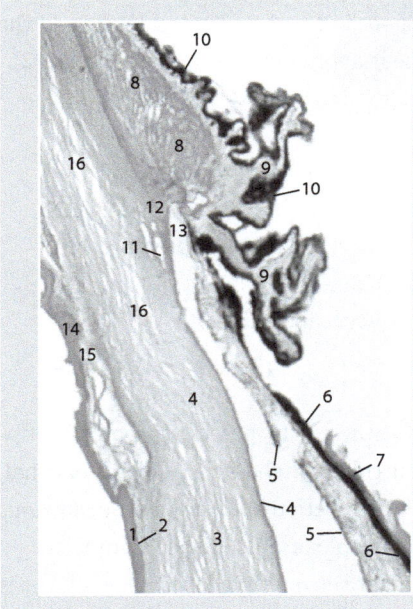

1. Epithelium of cornea
2. Bowman's layer of cornea
3. Substantia propria of cornea
4. Endothelium of cornea bordering the anterior chamber
5. Anterior border of iris
6. Posterior epithelium of iris
7. Fragment of lens attached to the iris
8. Ciliary body, pars plana
9. Ciliary processes (pars plicata)
10. Pigmented epithelium of the blind retina
11. Schlemm's canal
12. Pectinate ligament of iris (uveal trabecula)
13. Iridocorneal (drainage) angle
14. Conjunctiva
15. Episcleral tissue
16. Sclera

Figure 2.2 Cross section of the anterior segment of the normal eye, showing sites of normal aqueous outflow. Reproduced with permission from Csillag [1].

secrete substances against a concentration gradient. Active secretion is independent of pressure and accounts for the majority of aqueous production. Ultrafiltration is a pressure-dependent movement along a pressure gradient: in the ciliary processes, hydrostatic pressure differences between the capillary pressure and IOP favors movement of fluid into the eye; the oncotic gradient between the capillary and IOPs does not favor fluid movement. Diffusion is a passive process in which ions move across a membrane, according to charge and concentration.

Aqueous humor provides oxygen and nutrients to ocular tissues, and maintains the pressure and shape of the eye. Components of aqueous humor include a protein concentration around 1% of the level of plasma, antioxidants, such as ascorbate and glutathione, and certain cytokines, such as transforming growth factor-beta.

Aqueous humor is secreted into the posterior chamber from when it flows slowly through the pupil into the anterior chamber. The average rate of production of aqueous humor is 2.0–2.5 μL per minute, and the turnover rate for aqueous volume is approximately 1% per minute [2].

Aqueous humor outflow

There are two pathways for outflow of aqueous humor:

- the trabecular or conventional outflow pathway, through which most of the aqueous humor leaves the eye (this is pressure dependent [dependent on IOP]); and
- uveoscleral pathway (this is pressure independent).

Trabecular outflow pathway

Most of the aqueous humor leaves the eye by passing through the trabecular meshwork into a circular collector channel, Schlemm's canal, which is located at the corneoscleral junction and empties into aqueous veins in the scleral surface through a plexus of collector channels.

The trabecular meshwork comprises multiple layers. Each layer is composed of a collagenous connective tissue core covered by a continuous endothelial layer. Aqueous humor outflow via the trabecular meshwork is pressure-dependent and acts as a one-way valve, so that there is bulk flow of aqueous humor out of the eye but limited retrograde flow. Conventional outflow is passive. The point of maximum resistance to outflow is the juxtacanalicular trabecular meshwork (ie, the portion of trabecular meshwork closest to Schlemm's canal) and the inner wall of the canal itself.

The number of trabecular cells decreases with age, and the basement membrane thickens. In some eyes, the trabecular cells contain many pigment granules in the cytoplasm, thus giving the meshwork a brown appearance. Schlemm's canal is a single channel (average diameter of approximately 370 μm) that is traversed by tubules. The canal is connected to episcleral veins via a complex system of vessels. The episcleral veins drain into the anterior ciliary and superior ophthalmic veins, and these vessels drain into the cavernous sinus. Low IOP may be associated with collapse of the trabecular meshwork or blood reflux into Schlemm's canal.

Although blood may reflux into Schlemm's canal when the IOP is low, or episcleral venous pressure is high, the unidirectional nature of flow through trabecular meshwork prevents reflux into the anterior chamber [3].

Uveoscleral outflow pathway

Some aqueous humor exits through the root of the iris and the ciliary muscle into the suprachoroidal space. Low pressure in the suprachoroidal space provides a pressure gradient from the anterior chamber to this space, encouraging aqueous diffusion. Aqueous in the suprachoroidal space is absorbed through sclera into the connective tissue of the orbit, where it drains into blood vessels; some aqueous humor is directly absorbed by the blood vessels of the choroid.

This uveoscleral pathway provides an alternative route of aqueous absorption that can be modified pharmacologically to some degree (Figure 2.3). Although uveoscleral outflow follows a pressure gradient, it is largely pressure-independent, and is thought to comprise up to 15% of total aqueous humor outflow in humans, although this percentage varies greatly in other animals. Uveoscleral outflow is influenced by age and is increased by cycloplegia (ie, paralysis of the ciliary muscle of the eye), adrenergic agents, prostaglandin analogues and certain complications of surgery. It is decreased by miotics.

Outflow of aqueous humor through the uveoscleral pathway

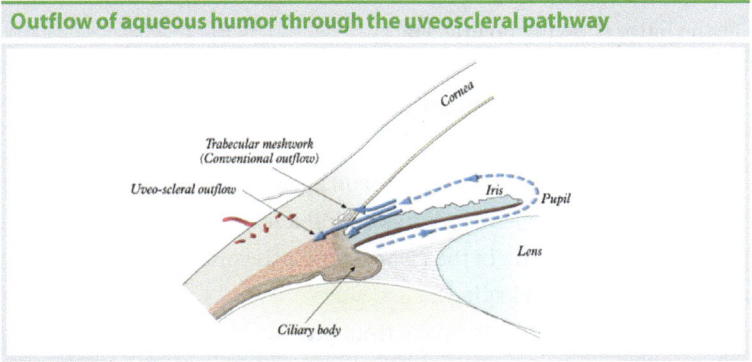

Figure 2.3 Outflow of aqueous humor through the uveoscleral pathway. Cross-section showing the normal flow of aqueous humor, but also illustrating both conventional outflow through the trabecular meshwork and uveoscleral outflow, which takes place via the root of the iris, ciliary body and suprachoroidal space. Courtesy of Alan Lacey, reproduced with permission from © Moorfields Eye Hospital, 2013. All Rights Reserved.

Disturbances in aqueous humor production and outflow

Aqueous humor is produced and circulates constantly, although there is a large variation between daytime (2–3 µl/min) [2] and nocturnal production, with the lowest levels occurring during sleep (approximately 1.4 µl/min) [4]. Various other factors influence the rate of aqueous humor production. These include:

- age;
- integrity of the blood–aqueous barrier;
- blood flow to the ciliary body (eg, reduced in carotid-occlusive disease);
- neurohormonal regulation of vascular tissue and the ciliary epithelium;
- detachment of the ciliary body (eg, after trauma);
- cyclitis or cyclitic membranes (eg, in intraocular inflammation);
- cyclophotocoagulation (eg, with the diode laser); and
- certain drugs (eg, general anesthetics, some systemic hypotensive agents).

The ratio of trabecular to uveoscleral outflow is affected by age and ocular health. Aqueous humor outflow facility varies greatly in healthy eyes and is affected by:

- age (although conflicting results have been found in cadaveric and in vivo studies, the former showing a reduction with increasing age, the latter showing no effect);
- trabecular cell function (influenced by corticosteroids) and ciliary muscle tone (influenced by cholinergic drugs);
- trauma;
- surgery (penetrating keratoplasty and aphakia may result in distortion of the trabecular meshwork spaces, influencing outflow facility);
- extracellular matrix in the trabecular meshwork (affected by corticosteroids and aging);
- trabecular meshwork damage from prolonged or severe IOP elevation; and
- angle occlusion (eg, primary angle-closure glaucoma [PACG] or neovascularization).

Impact of aqueous flow on intraocular pressure

The IOP is determined by the modified Goldmann equation (see Table 2.1), which relates the various components of inflow and outflow. It can be seen by this equation that a balance between the production (aqueous flow) and outflow determines the IOP (Table 2.2). Although aqueous flow declines with age [1], the influence of age on IOP has been less clear. Cross-sectional studies have not shown a consistent trend. One recent longitudinal study followed 339 individuals in Northern Sweden for 21 years and reported a small but significant increase in IOP of 0.05 mmHg per year in IOP [5]. An increase in outflow resistance with age has an important influence on IOP stability. The impact on IOP of a small change in aqueous flow will have a large effect on IOP if the facility of outflow is low (high outflow resistance), but less so if the facility of outflow is large (eg, as in the case of young, healthy individuals). The most common cause of IOP elevation in eyes with open angles is inadequate drainage (ie, reduced outflow) of aqueous humor due to increased resistance in the trabecular meshwork.

Modified Goldmann equation	
Equation	**Components**
	IOP, intraocular pressure
	Fa, aqueous flow
$IOP=(Fa-Fu)/C+Pev$	Fu, uveoscleral outflow
	C, facility of outflow
	Pev, episcleral venous pressure

Table 2.1 Modified Goldmann equation. As IOP can be directly measured and uveoscleral outflow cannot, this equation is usually used to calculate the latter.

Production and outflow of aqueous humor and intraocular pressure		
Outflow facility	**Change in aqueous flow**	**Change in IOP**
High outflow (eg, in young healthy individuals)	Small increase	Small increase
Low outflow (eg, in glaucoma sufferers)	Small increase	Disproportionate increase

Table 2.2 Production and outflow of aqueous humor and intraocular pressure. A small change in aqueous flow can produce a larger change in pressure, depending on facility of outflow. IOP, intraocular pressure.

Mechanisms of intraocular pressure disturbance in glaucoma

Primary open-angle glaucoma

The anterior chamber angle, by definition, is normal in primary open-angle glaucoma (POAG) and there is no evidence of iridotrabecular contact (Figure 2.4) [3]. The reduced outflow of aqueous humor in POAG is caused by reduction in the function of the trabecular meshwork, raising IOP.

Angle closure glaucoma

In angle-closure glaucoma, aqueous does not reach the trabecular meshwork because access to the anterior chamber angle is obstructed by the iris (in primary angle-closure) or sometimes other tissues (some secondary glaucomas), leading to elevated IOP levels (Figure 2.5). Angle closure is deemed to have occurred when the iris is in contact with the trabecular meshwork over part or the entire circumference of the anterior chamber angle. Angle closure may be due to intermittent apposition and, therefore, may be reversible (appositional), although prolonged iridotrabecular contact results in adhesions (synechia), and irreversible angle closure.

Angle closure may occur as a result of several possible mechanisms, both primary and secondary. Primary angle-closure is defined as

Diagram of open-angle glaucoma

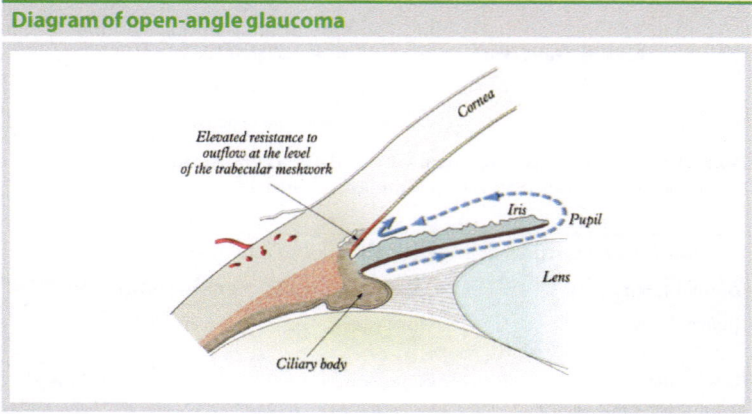

Figure 2.4 Diagram of open-angle glaucoma. When the intraocular pressure is elevated in primary open-angle glaucoma, the iridocorneal angle is anatomically open, but aqueous humor fails to drain through the trabecular meshwork to Schlemm's canal at a sufficient rate. Evidence suggests that facility of outflow reduces with age (ie, that trabecular meshwork resistance increases). The point of maximum resistance seems to be around the juxtacanalicular trabecular meshwork. Courtesy of Alan Lacey, reproduced with permission from © Moorfields Eye Hospital, 2013. All Rights Reserved.

Diagram of angle-closure glaucoma (pupillary block)

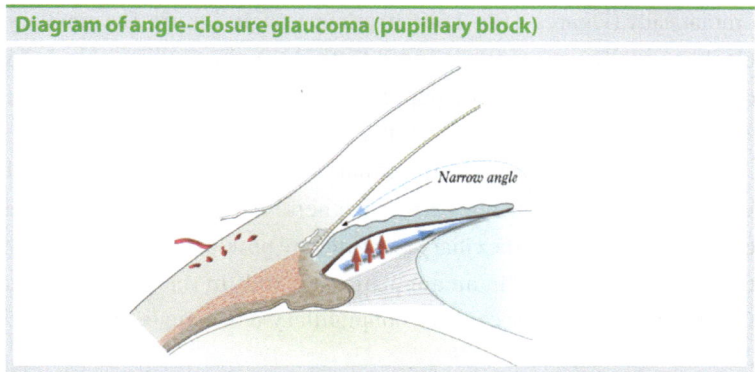

Narrow angle

Figure 2.5 Diagram of angle-closure glaucoma (pupillary block). Diagrammatic representation of angle closure secondary to pupillary block. As a result of elevated resistance to aqueous flow between the front of the lens and the pupillary margin, aqueous pressure behind the mid-periphery of the iris exceeds that in front, the iris balloons forward (arrows) and obstructs the trabecular meshwork, further presenting aqueous outflow. Courtesy of Alan Lacey, reproduced with permission from © Moorfields Eye Hospital, 2013. All Rights Reserved.

iridotrabecular apposition with or without IOP elevation or peripheral anterior synechia. PACG is diagnosed only in the presence of concurrent glaucomatous optic neuropathy (GON) in addition to iridotrabecular apposition. In cases where the optic nerve cannot be visualized, the diagnosis of PACG can be made in the presence of a closed angle if the IOP is above the 99.5% for the normal population (around 27 mmHg) [6].

The most common mechanism of primary angle-closure is pupillary block (Figures 2.5, 2.6), in which a relative obstruction to flow occurs as aqueous passes from the posterior to anterior chamber. Pupillary block usually develops in eyes that are predisposed in that they are anatomically small and hypermetropic with some constitutional narrowing of the drainage angle. Often, with increasing age, an increase in the anteroposterior thickness of the crystalline lens induces pupillary block in an eye that already has a slightly narrow angle.

Pupillary block develops when the anterior lens surface comes into contact with the pupil margin thereby obstructing the forward passage of aqueous humor from the posterior to the anterior chambers (Figure 2.5). This resultant pressure differential causes the mid-section of the iris to "balloon" forward (iris bombé), occluding the trabecular meshwork, further obstructing aqueous outflow and elevating the pressure dramatically (Figures 2.6A, 2.6B). In primary angle-closure, the pupillary block is usually not complete and is termed *relative* pupillary block, in contradistinction to *absolute* pupillary block that sometimes occurs in secondary glaucomas, such as uveitis (see Figure 1.7).

In a proportion of eyes with primary angle-closure, an anatomical variation in the ciliary body and peripheral iris profile causes angle closure. In plateau iris, the ciliary processes are positioned more anteriorly than normal, resulting in an angulation or "roll" in the peripheral iris (Figure 2.6C). In other cases of nonpupillary block angle closure, the

Angle closure from pupillary block on anterior segment optical coherence tomography

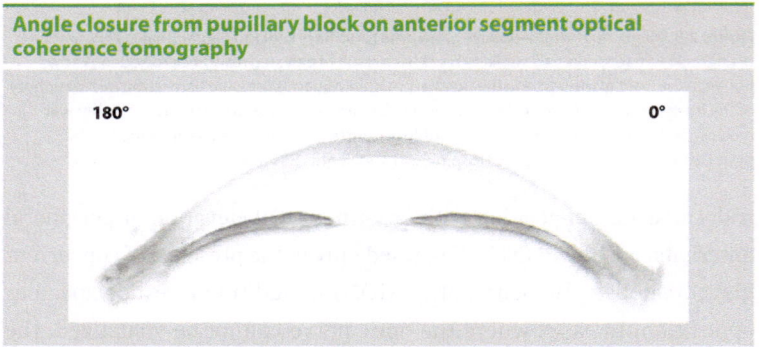

Figure 2.6A Angle closure from pupillary block on anterior segment optical coherence tomography. Note the convexity of the peripheral iris, which is the hallmark of pupillary block. Compare this with the flat iris plane in Figure 2.6B below. Reproduced with permission from © Moorfields Eye Hospital, 2013. All Rights Reserved.

Normal angle on anterior segment optical coherence tomography for comparison

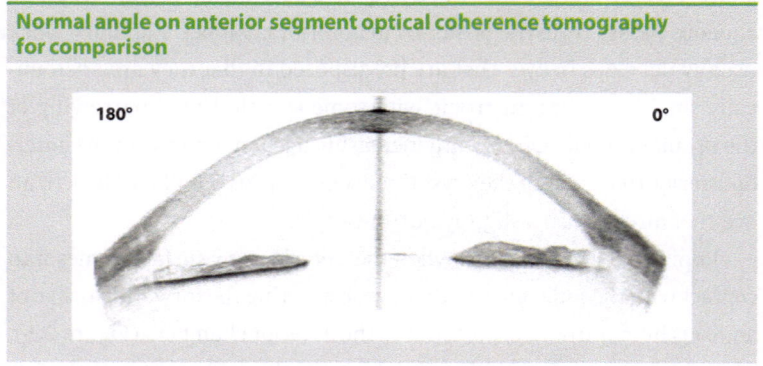

Figure 2.6B Normal angle on anterior segment optical coherence tomography for comparison. Reproduced with permission from © Moorfields Eye Hospital, 2013. All Rights Reserved.

iris root is inserted in the anterior face of the ciliary body. On pupillary dilation, either at night or pharmacologically, the peripheral iris obstructs the trabecular meshwork. While ultrasound biomicroscopy is necessary to differentiate these two variants, functionally they cause angle closure by the same mechanism.

Typically, they cause angle closure without pupillary block; however, with modern imaging techniques, an element of pupillary block is often also detected. Laser iridotomy is often performed to exclude pupillary block and make the diagnosis of plateau iris, but will often not prevent recurrent angle closure.

In chronic primary angle-closure (CPAC), chronic iridotrabecular contact results in permanent iridotrabecular adhesions, chronic IOP elevation and eventually GON. At this time CPAC becomes chronic primary angle-closure glaucoma (CPACG).

Secondary glaucoma

In secondary glaucoma, drainage is impaired as a result of trabecular meshwork obstruction (eg, secondary angle closure in neovascular glaucoma), direct trauma to the iridocorneal angle (traumatic glaucoma) or reduced trabecular meshwork function (eg, secondary open-angle glaucoma following chronic corticosteroid usage). Certain conditions, such as uveitis, may cause IOP elevation via a mixture of these mechanisms.

A narrow angle in an eye without pupillary block

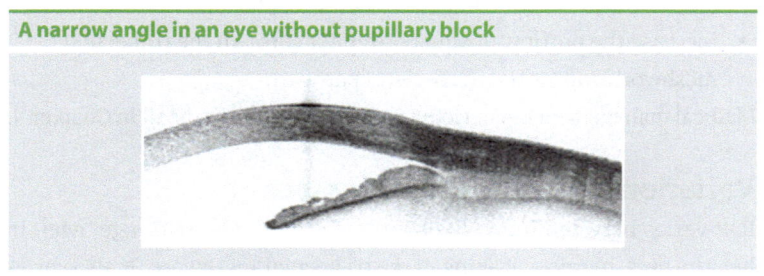

Figure 2.6C A narrow angle in an eye without pupillary block. In this high-resolution optical coherence tomography example the root of the iris can be seen originating from the anterior face of the ciliary body, creating a prominent bulge in the peripheral iris, which is consequently thicker than the mid-periphery, potentially occluding the angle when the pupil dilates. In a proportion of such cases ultrasound biomicroscopy would show loss of the iridociliary sulcus, the hallmark of plateau iris syndrome. Reproduced with permission from © Moorfields Eye Hospital, 2013. All Rights Reserved.

Impact of elevated intraocular pressure on the eye

Elevated IOP adversely influences the health of intraocular tissues in a number of ways:

- Mechanical damage to the optic nerve as it passes through the lamina cribrosa:
  - The structural integrity of the lamina cribrosa is believed to be important for the long-term health of the RGC axons passing out of the eye at this, the weakest point, in the scleral wall of the eye. Laminar distortion at the optic disc may disrupt both orthograde and retrograde axoplasmic flow. This in turn reduces the integrity and ultimately the health of the RGC.
  - Direct pressure on RGC axons may also be important in eyes with very high pressure.
- Elevated IOP also reduces ocular perfusion, compromises RGC nutrition and impedes axonal transport within RGC axons.

If IOP is sufficiently elevated, it may also damage other tissues within the eye. For example, glaucoma has been implicated in retinal vein occlusion, and protracted high IOP elevation also results in increased corneal endothelial cell loss and lens opacification.

All currently available drugs for treating glaucoma act by lowering the IOP via one or both of the following mechanisms:

- reduce the production of aqueous humor; and/or
- increase the outflow of aqueous humor through the trabecular meshwork and/or the uveoscleral pathway.

Medical management of glaucoma is discussed in more detail in Chapter 4.

Variations in intraocular pressure

IOP varies between individuals and rises gradually with age, even in healthy eyes, because of aging of the trabecular meshwork. It also varies diurnally, as discussed below and in Chapter 3.

Because IOP elevation is the most important modifiable risk factor for glaucoma, accurate measurement of IOP by tonometry is paramount in diagnosing and monitoring the progression of glaucoma. Tonometry is discussed in more detail in Chapter 3.

Intraocular pressure threshold for glaucoma

A number of studies, such as the Advanced Glaucoma Intervention Study, have helped characterize the relationship between deterioration of visual field and IOP. Although, there seems to be no *fixed* IOP threshold above which glaucoma develops, an arbitrary divide between normal and high IOP has been defined as 21 mmHg because this represents two standard deviations above the mean IOP in an adult Caucasian population (see Figure 1.8). This was based on a clinical assumption that glaucomatous damage occurred only when IOP was raised, as normal tension glaucoma (NTG) was not recognized at that time. It is now clear that screening for glaucoma based solely on IOP >21 mmHg would fail to identify almost half of the individuals with glaucoma, so this criterion is no longer used to determine who needs therapy. The current consensus is that there is no clear IOP level below which pressure can be considered normal or safe, although the risk of progression seems to be very low over in individuals whose pressure is consistently in the lower part of the normal range [7].

Although several other risk factors may affect an individual's susceptibility to glaucomatous damage, IOP is currently the only one that can be effectively modified. The use of IOP targets in monitoring glaucoma management is discussed in Chapter 4.

Circadian fluctuations in intraocular pressure

IOP fluctuates over a 24-hour period (circadian fluctuation) as well as during the day (diurnal fluctuation). Circadian fluctuation in healthy eyes is less (usually 2–6 mmHg) than in eyes with glaucoma, and it has been suggested in the past that fluctuation greater than 10 mmHg is indicative of glaucoma. IOP levels can vary enormously during the day and night, and are influenced by many factors including:

- time of day;
- heartbeat;
- respiration;
- exercise;
- fluid intake;
- systemic and topical medications;

- position (recumbent or upright); and
- activities, such as diving, playing wind instruments.

In a study of 64 patients with POAG who measured their own IOP 5 times daily for 5 days using home tonometry, the range of fluctuation in IOP in one day and over multiple days were both significant independent risk factors for progression of glaucoma [8]. The nature and extent of the fluctuation, including the time at which peak IOP occur, vary between individuals; however, many individuals reach peak daytime pressures in the early morning hours while they are still in bed [9]. In this study, IOP fluctuation outside office hours was a significant risk factor for progression independent of IOP measured in the office. The study led to the concept that IOP fluctuation might be a risk factor for progression, independent of the level of IOP; however, in one study that seemed to support this hypothesis, fluctuation was not independent of mean IOP and, therefore, was not an independent risk factor [10]. In another study–a population-based randomized clinical trial of therapy for glaucoma–there was no correlation between fluctuation and progression [11].

The current consensus is that a single measurement of IOP is insufficient to identify peak IOP or mean diurnal pressure. Measurement at more than one time of day may be required if patients appear to be progressing when the IOP appears satisfactory during routine office examination. This is discussed in more detail in Chapter 3.

Ocular blood flow and glaucoma

The role of ocular, or optic nerve, blood flow in the pathogenesis of glaucoma is unclear. Given that a significant proportion of patients have NTG, and that progression of glaucoma is, not uncommonly, characterized by hemorrhages in the retinal nerve fiber layer around the optic disc [12], it seems likely that factors other than raised IOP contribute to glaucomatous optic nerve damage. For over 100 years ischemia has been thought to be one such factor; however, the exact role of vascular changes in optic nerve head disease remains unclear.

Ocular blood flow depends on both perfusion pressure (blood pressure minus IOP) and resistance to flow within the arterioles and capillary bed. A number of epidemiological studies have shown that low diastolic blood pressure and low diastolic ocular perfusion pressure (DOPP) are associated with an increased prevalence of POAG; for example, a DOPP of less than 30 mmHg has been reported to be associated with a sixfold increase in risk of POAG [13]. The average DOPP was 53 mmHg for subjects with POAG compared with 63 mmHg for those without in the Barbados Eye Study [14]. Low ocular perfusion pressure has also been associated with increased progression of glaucoma [15]. An area of concern has been low nocturnal systemic blood pressure, or *nocturnal dipping*, in systemic blood pressure [15]. This is believed to be an issue particularly in patients with systemic hypertension who are treated aggressively.

A number of techniques exist to measure ocular blood flow (Table 2.3) [16]. These have demonstrated reduced flow in patients with glaucoma.

Methods of measuring ocular blood flow		
Technique	**Measurement made**	**Notes**
Scanning laser ophthalmoscopic angiography	With fluorescein, to measure arteriovenous passage time; with indocyanine green dye, to measure speed of blood flow entering the choroid	Superior to photographic angiography because the laser beam gives better penetration of the lens and cornea. Indocyanine green dye uses near infrared light, which penetrates retinal layers better than shorter wavelengths used with fluorescein
Confocal scanning laser Doppler flowmetry	Combines a flow meter to measure speed of blood and confocal scanning laser tomography taking images of the optic nerve head and retina	Reproducibility over time is limited
Ocular pulse measurement	Calculates flow from pulsation in the IOP during the cardiac cycle	Affected by sclera rigidity, ocular volume, heart rate, systemic blood pressure and IOP, limiting its usefulness for comparison between individuals, but not for following blood flow in a single patient. More suitable for measuring blood flow changes in an individual (eg, in response to medication) than comparisons between individuals (eg, glaucoma versus normal). Fast and easy to use, relatively inexpensive
Color Doppler ultrasound imaging	Grayscale image of anatomical details is combined with color representation of blood flow measured by Doppler shift	Absolute volume of flow not measured because vessel diameter is not measured

Table 2.3 Methods of measuring ocular blood flow. IOP, intraocular pressure. Adapted from Flammer [16].

For example, color Doppler imaging has shown increased resistance to flow in POAG [17] and NTG [18], and reduction in blood flow in the temporal neuroretinal rim, and the cup of the optic nerve head has been demonstrated by scanning laser Doppler flowmetry [19]; however, the relevance of this to clinical practice has not been determined.

References

1   Csillag A. The organ of vision. In: *Atlas of the Sensory Organs: Functional and Clinical Anatomy*. New York, NY: Springer-Verlag, LLC; 2005:85-164.

2   Brubaker RF. Flow of aqueous humor in humans [The Friedenwald Lecture]. *Invest Ophthalmol Vis Sci*. 1991;32:3145-3166.

3   American Academy of Ophthalmology: The Eye M.D. Association. In: *2011-2012 Basic and Clinical Science Course, Section 10: Glaucoma*. San Francisco, CA: American Academy of Ophthalmology; 2011.

4   Reiss GR, Lee DA, Topper JE, Brubaker RF. Aqueous humor flow during sleep. *Invest Ophthalmol Vis Sci*. 1984;25:776-778.

5   Astrom S, Stenlund H, Linden C. Intraocular pressure changes over 21 years - a longitudinal age-cohort study in northern Sweden. *Acta Ophthalmol*. 2013 Jul 31. [Epub ahead of print].

6   Foster PJ, Buhrmann R, Quigley HA, et al. The definition and classification of glaucoma in prevalence surveys. *Br J Ophthalmol*. 2002;86:238-244.

7   The Advanced Glaucoma Intervention Study (AGIS): 7. The relationship between control of intraocular pressure and visual field deterioration. The AGIS Investigators. *Am J Ophthalmol*. 2000;130:429-440.

8   Asrani S, Zeimer R, Wilensky J, et al. Large diurnal fluctuations in intraocular pressure are an independent risk factor in patients with glaucoma. *J Glaucoma*. 2000;9:134-142.

9   Barkana Y, Anis S, Liebmann J, et al. Clinical utility of intraocular pressure monitoring outside of normal office hours in patients with glaucoma. *Arch Ophthalmol*. 2006;124:793-797.

10 Nouri-Madhavi K, Hoffman D, Coleman AL, et al. Predictive factors for glaucomatous visual field progression in the Advanced Glaucoma Intervention Study. *Ophthalmology*. 2004;111:1627-1635.

11 Bengtsson B, Leske MC, Hyman L, et al. Fluctuation of intraocular pressure and glaucoma progression in the early manifest glaucoma trial. *Ophthalmology*. 2007;114:205-209.

12 Leske MC, Heijl A, Hyman L, et al. Predictors of long-term progression in the early manifest glaucoma trial. *Ophthalmology*. 2007;114:1965-1972.

13 Tielsch JM, Katz J, Sommer A. Hypertension, perfusion pressure, and primary open-angle glaucoma. A population-based assessment. *Arch Ophthalmol*. 1995;113:216-221.

14 Leske MC, Connell AM, Wu SY, et al. Risk factors for open-angle glaucoma. The Barbados Eye Study. *Arch Ophthalmol*. 1995;113:918-924.

15 Graham SL, Drance SM, Wijsman K, et al. Ambulatory blood pressure monitoring in glaucoma. The nocturnal dip. *Ophthalmology*. 1995;102:61-69.

16 Flammer J. *Glaucoma: a guide for patients*. 3rd edition. Bern, Switzerland: Hogrefe & Huber; 2006.

17 Rankin SJ, Walman BE, Buckley AR, et al. Color Doppler imaging and spectral analysis of the optic nerve vasculature in glaucoma. *Am J Ophthalmol*. 1995;119:685-693.

18 Harris A, Sergott RC, Spaeth GL, et al. Color Doppler analysis of ocular vessel blood velocity in normal-tension glaucoma. *Am J Ophthalmol*. 1994;118:642-649.

19 Fuchsjäger-Mayrl G, Wally B, Georgopoulos M, et al. Ocular blood flow and systemic blood pressure in patients with primary open-angle glaucoma and ocular hypertension. *Invest Ophthalmol Vis Sci*. 2004;45:834-839.

Chapter 3

Diagnosing glaucoma

Early detection and accurate diagnosis of glaucoma are vital if treatment is to be initiated early in the course of the disease at a stage when treatment is probably easiest and most effective, thereby reducing the risk of severe vision loss or blindness. As mentioned in Chapter 1, there is no single screening test for glaucoma, and no single test that makes the diagnosis. The diagnosis of glaucoma is a clinical judgment, based on the collective evidence obtained from a careful patient history, the results of a number of evaluation techniques, including quantitative measurement of visual field defects, of intraocular pressure (IOP) and the visible appearance of the retina and optic disc. For example, angle narrowing and closure is suspected on clinical examination from the patient's refraction (most are hypermetropic) from shallowing of the anterior chamber, especially the peripheral anterior chamber (van Herick method), on slit-lamp biomicroscopy and on gonioscopy.

Where underlying systemic disease is suspected and further systemic testing or examination is required, it may be necessary to refer the patient to a specialist in the relevant field.

History

The history should cover:
- Symptoms: as primary open-angle glaucoma (POAG) is usually asymptomatic unless diagnosed late, few patients notice visual loss at presentation. Nevertheless, some patients may notice a positive scotoma if the first visual field defect develops close to fixation.

K. Barton and R. A. Hitchings, *Medical Management of Glaucoma*, 49
DOI: 10.1007/978-1-907673-44-3_3, © Springer Healthcare 2013

- Previous ophthalmic problems, such as myopia, eye injuries, contact lens wear and especially prior refractive surgery or other ocular surgery.
- Previous systemic problems, especially cardiovascular or pulmonary disease, diabetes, hypertension, migraines, Raynaud's phenomenon (particularly cold hands or feet) or other serious illnesses. It is important to elicit a history of asthma or chest disease as this may limit the use of beta-blockers if treatment is required. Rarely, patients with severe asthma or other chronic chest disease may require long courses of systemic corticosteroids that occasionally elevate the IOP.
- Current medications and a history of allergy to medications: a full drug history is essential to elicit as a number of systemic medications may exacerbate glaucoma, especially anticholinergics and antihistamines.
- Family history of glaucoma, especially in first-degree relatives. In those with a number of first-degree relatives affected, it is also helpful to know how many are unaffected.

Overview of assessments used in the diagnosis of glaucoma

A careful clinical examination is essential when making the diagnosis of glaucoma and this should include:

- measurement of the visual acuity;
- assessment of the pupillary responses;
- measurement of the central corneal thickness (CCT) (pachymetry);
- slit-lamp biomicroscopy;
- measurement of the IOP;
- careful gonioscopy to examine the angle in all patients;
- dilated fundus examination to document the appearance of the optic nerve head and nerve fiber layer; and
- assessment of the visual field.

The best corrected Snellen visual acuity and visual field testing are usually performed before other aspects of the clinical examination. Extremes of refractive error (ie, high myopia or hypermetropia) are noted as these extremes increase the risk of glaucoma. The pupillary responses are then examined to detect the presence of an afferent pupillary defect. Corneal pachymetry is best performed before gonioscopy and is often most conveniently measured before slit-lamp examination. IOP is usually measured before gonioscopy, and the pupils should not be dilated until gonioscopy has been performed.

Pachymetry

Measurement of CCT is an important part of the examination of all new patients presenting with a suspicion of ocular hypertension (OHT) or glaucoma, as it influences the accuracy of IOP estimation. There are numerous methods of measuring the CCT. Optical pachymetry, which utilizes a slit-lamp based device, is rarely performed today as ultrasound pachymeters are much more convenient. In addition, there are a number of newer optical methods of measuring CCT, including anterior segment optical coherence tomography.

Normal CCT is 530–545 nm [1]. Increased CCT can lead to an over-estimation of IOP, and reduced CCT, an underestimation. An exception to this is in eyes that have corneal edema where a thick cornea can be compatible with an under-reading of the CCT. In OHT, of the various baseline factors predicting conversion to POAG, there appeared to be an association between CCT and risk of conversion [2]. This was suspected to have resulted from a number of trial patients with presumed OHT, who in reality only had thicker than average CCT rather than true OHT. These individuals were clearly not at risk of conversion to glaucoma. Although CCT was not initially found to be an independent risk factor for progression of glaucoma in the Early Manifest Glaucoma Trial after 5 years of follow-up [3], longer term analysis, with up to 11 years of follow-up, CCT was reported to be an independent risk factor [4].

An elevated CCT might therefore increase the risk of receiving an inappropriate diagnosis of OHT, but a low CCT appears to be a risk factor for glaucoma. The role of CCT in OHT is perhaps less important than its role in assessing the risk of progression at a given IOP level for patients with manifest glaucoma. In the Early Manifest Glaucoma Trial [3], the higher risk of progression in patients with thinner corneas was only seen in those with higher IOP levels, indicating that either thinner CCT is an adjunctive risk factor to higher IOP, or those who progressed had even higher IOP than that documented; this was masked by thinner CCT so that the patients were less aggressively treated than otherwise might have been the case.

CCT appears to reduce very slightly with age, is slightly lower in females than males, and in certain races (eg, Mongolians, Japanese and West Africans) seems to have lower CCT than others (eg, Caucasians, Hispanics, Chinese and Koreans).

Slit-lamp examination

On slit-lamp examination the cornea and anterior chambers are examined for signs of primary angle-closure and secondary causes of glaucoma. The anterior chamber depth is documented. If the central anterior chamber depth is less than threefold the CCT, the eye is deemed to be at a higher risk of angle closure. Although the risk of angle closure is lower when the central anterior is more than threefold the CCT, a significant proportion of cases of angle closure still occur in this group.

The peripheral or limbal anterior chamber depth can be estimated by setting the slit-beam perpendicular to the temporal limbal cornea and viewing at an angle of 60 degrees (Figure 3.1). The limbal anterior chamber

Assessment of limbal anterior chamber depth, modified van Herick test

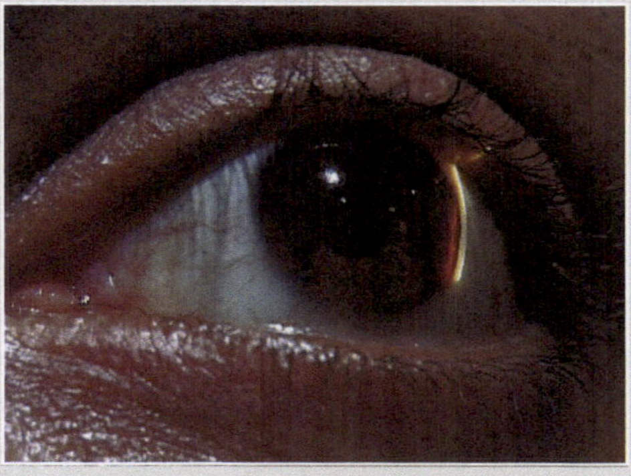

Figure 3.1 Assessment of limbal anterior chamber depth, modified van Herick test.
Reproduced with permission from © Moorfields Eye Hospital, 2013. All Rights Reserved.

depth is then seen as the gap between the posterior corneal surface and the peripheral iris. This technique was described by van Herick [4], and has been validated by Foster [5]; however, accurate assessment of the limbal anterior chamber depth, like gonioscopy, requires experience and should therefore be performed regularly.

Tonometry

Arguably the simplest way to detect glaucoma is to measure the IOP. If the IOP is elevated, then the individual should be examined fully for glaucoma; however, it must be remembered that measuring IOP alone will miss around 50% of patients with glaucoma.

Measurement technique

IOP is usually measured before gonioscopy, and the standard method of measurement uses Goldmann applanation tonometry (GAT). GAT is a contact method, requiring corneal anesthesia. The tonometer calibration should be checked regularly. The technique is described in detail elsewhere but a few points are worth noting. Firstly the examiner must ensure that the corneal meniscus is thin (Figure 3.2) in order to optimize the accuracy of the reading.

More than one reading should be taken from each eye and ideally the tonometer gauge reset to zero or to another random number between measurements.

The results of tonometry are influenced by corneal biomechanics, most notably by CCT (see above) but probably also by other factors that are as yet not measured in routine clinical practice.

Although GAT remains the *gold standard* for IOP measurement in clinical practice, a number of new devices are now available that offer other benefits. A number of noncontact devices exist, including the ocular response analyzer (ORA) (Reichert Corporation). The ORA is noteworthy because it gives additional information with regard to corneal biomechanical properties than IOP alone, though the IOP readings obtained are affected to a greater extent by CCT than GAT readings. At the time of writing, the dynamic contour tonometer (Swiss Microtechnology AG), a contact device incorporating a pressure sensor into a tip that matches

Goldmann applanation tonometry, demonstrating thin Menisci

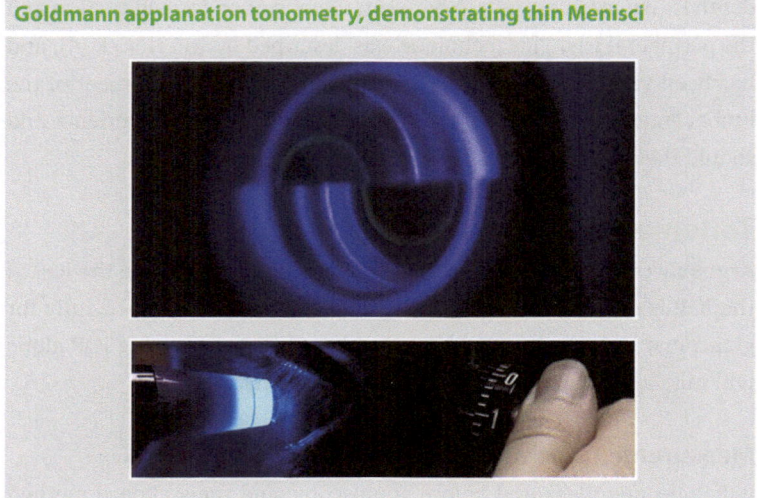

Figure 3.2 Goldmann applanation tonometry, demonstrating thin Menisci. Reproduced with permission from © Moorfields Eye Hospital, 2013. All Rights Reserved.

the contour of the eye, has been reported to offer similar accuracy and precision to GAT, but is less influenced by corneal thickness.

Repeat measurement of intraocular pressure

Given the variation of IOP with time of day and other factors (see Chapter 2) for any one patient, serial measurement of IOP is required when assessing patients with glaucoma or suspected glaucoma.

Monitoring intraocular pressure for twenty-four hours

It is important to remember that measurements of IOP in the clinic represent a mere snapshot of the pressure profile and that IOP varies enormously; a large diurnal IOP range is generally believed to be a risk factor for glaucoma [6]. Monitoring for 24 hours has not been widespread because it is inconvenient for the patient and logistically difficult in the day-care setting; however, there are instances when it may be important to measure the pressure at different times of the day in order to establish the range of diurnal fluctuation or even overnight to gain a more accurate impression of the circadian curve in a particular patient (eg, when glaucoma is progressing despite apparently normal IOP levels).

While diurnal measurement is relatively straightforward to organize, overnight measurement is rather more difficult. Circumstances in which this might be done are those where glaucoma is progressing unexpectedly in the absence of IOP elevation during office hours, especially in patients with significant visual field loss.

Demonstration of IOP elevation outside office hours can influence treatment as more aggressive treatment may be required if a patient is exhibiting a peak pressure outside office hours; however, arguably the value of overnight measurement is limited as patients demonstrated progress at any particular office pressure level should be treated more aggressively anyway. Demonstration of a high-peak outside office hours may be useful in those progressing at apparently low IOP levels as this visible demonstration of a high IOP level can be useful in justifying the need for more aggressive treatment, such as surgery, to the patient.

It is also true that different topical medications vary in the time course of their IOP-lowering effect, and sometimes a high nocturnal IOP measurement may influence medical treatment. This has been observed in at least two studies. In one retrospective study of 22 patients with POAG admitted for 24-hour monitoring, higher peak IOPs were observed outside office hours than had previously been observed during office visits in 69% of subjects as well as significantly higher mean IOP fluctuation than that during office hours (6.9 +/- 2.9 mmHg versus 3.8 +/- 2.3 mmHg, $P<0.001$). Monitoring for 24 hours led to an alteration in treatment in 36% of the patients [7]. Similarly, a retrospective analysis of glaucoma patients admitted for 24-hour monitoring found that peak IOP levels occurred outside office hours in just over half of 29 patients, requiring a change in management in 23 (79.3%), including surgery in 13 (45%) [8].

These findings that are of interest, but must be taken in the context that both were retrospective studies of patients selected for 24-hour monitoring and, therefore, are likely to be those identified as progressing or at higher risk of progression; consequently, they are likely to have undergone a change in therapy even if these higher measurements were not obtained. Although 24-hour monitoring is likely to be helpful, its full value in clinical practice is still not completely certain.

Gonioscopy

Gonioscopy is performed on slit-lamp examination using a contact lens incorporating a prism (gonioprism) that overcomes internal reflection from the cornea, thereby allowing the observer to visualize the iridocorneal (anterior chamber) angle. Even though angle width can be easily imaged by modern noncontact devices, such as anterior segment optical coherence tomography (see Figure 2.6A for examples), gonioscopy remains the gold standard for angle assessment because other imaging techniques cannot accurately identify other angle abnormalities, such as synechia, pigment, neovascularization and iris processes.

It is possible to identify a wide range of abnormalities of the angle using gonioscopy. These include iris adhesions to the trabecular meshwork (peripheral anterior synechia), pigmentation of the trabecular meshwork, signs of intermittent iridotrabecular contact, new vessels, and traumatic damage to the drainage angle (angle recession and cyclodialysis clefts) as well as congenital anomalies, such as Axenfeld-Rieger syndrome. For example, in intermittent angle-closure glaucoma, narrowing of the iridocorneal angle will be found and there may be other suspicious features, such as iris pigment smudging on angle structures, a convex iris surface or plateau configuration of the peripheral iris, or even peripheral anterior synechia.

Angle narrowing can be detected and a distinction made between open angle and angle closure glaucoma. A consensus definition of an occludable angle is one in which the posterior trabecular meshwork can be visualized on gonioscopy for less than 90 degrees of the circumference of the drainage angle [9]. Information useful in ascertaining the type of angle closure can be gleaned. Gonioscopy is, therefore, an essential component in the diagnosis of any patient with elevated IOP and if glaucoma is suspected in a patient with normal IOP. Gonioscopy requires topical corneal anesthesia. Goldmann-type (nonindentation) gonio lenses also require coupling fluid, such as artificial tears or other viscous fluid.

There are two main types of gonioscopy: direct and indirect (Figure 3.3) [10].

Direct gonioscopy

Direct gonioscopy is a technique performed in the operating theater to examine the angle during surgery, primarily in cases of congenital glaucoma undergoing goniotomy, but may also be used to visualize other angle abnormalities intra-operatively if need be. With this technique, the angle is viewed directly using an operating theater microscope. Direct gonioscopy is not usually used in the diagnosis of glaucoma, except in young children undergoing examination under anesthesia where slit-lamp gonioscopy is impossible.

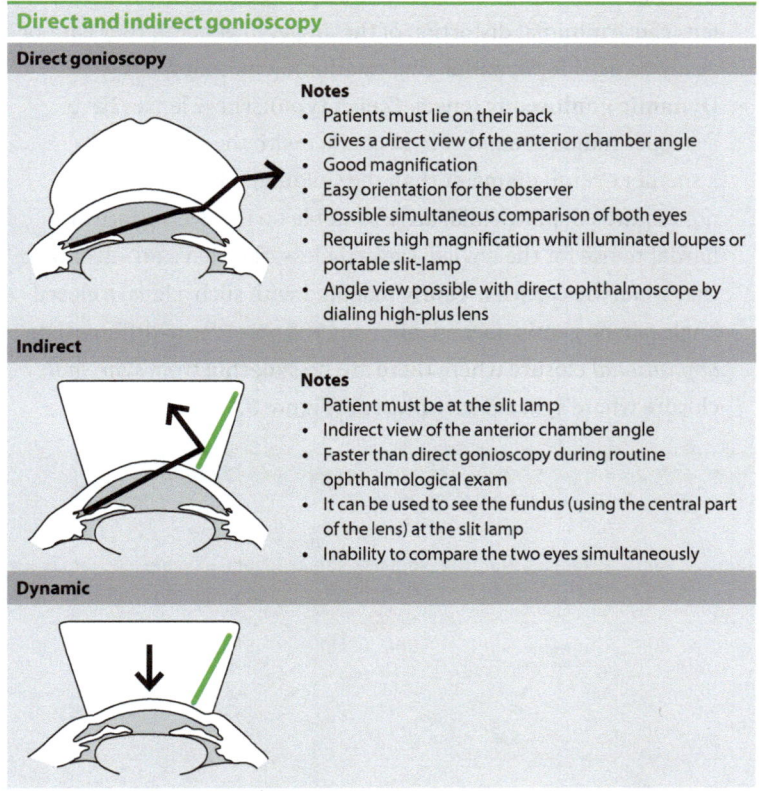

Direct and indirect gonioscopy

Direct gonioscopy

Notes
- Patients must lie on their back
- Gives a direct view of the anterior chamber angle
- Good magnification
- Easy orientation for the observer
- Possible simultaneous comparison of both eyes
- Requires high magnification whit illuminated loupes or portable slit-lamp
- Angle view possible with direct ophthalmoscope by dialing high-plus lens

Indirect

Notes
- Patient must be at the slit lamp
- Indirect view of the anterior chamber angle
- Faster than direct gonioscopy during routine ophthalmological exam
- It can be used to see the fundus (using the central part of the lens) at the slit lamp
- Inability to compare the two eyes simultaneously

Dynamic

Figure 3.3 Direct and indirect gonioscopy. Gonioscopic lenses eliminate the tear–air interface and total internal reflection. With a direct lens, the light ray reflected from the anterior chamber angle is observed directly, whereas with an indirect lens the light ray is reflected by a mirror within the lens. Posterior pressure with an indirect lens forces open an appositionally closed or narrow anterior chamber angle (dynamic gonioscopy). Reproduced with permission from © European Glaucoma Society, 2013 [10]. All Rights Reserved.

Indirect gonioscopy

This is the standard method of gonioscopy used at the slit lamp in the diagnosis of open or closed angle glaucoma. With indirect gonioscopy, the angle is viewed as a reflection by a mirror within the lens, usually of the portion of the angle 180 degrees away from the mirror.

There are a number of types of indirect gonio lens, falling into two categories:

- **Goldmann-type lenses:** these are often considered to be relatively easy to use. They require coupling fluid, but are very stable on the eye for the inexperienced ophthalmologist. These types of lens cause minimal distortion of the angle. In general, they cannot easily be used for dynamic (indentation) gonioscopy.

- **Dynamic gonioscopy lenses (Zeiss-type):** These lenses have a steeper radius of curvature in contact with the cornea and a smaller overall diameter than the Goldmann lenses. They do not require coupling fluid, are less stable on the eye surface and harder to use for the novice. Nevertheless, they have an advantage that when the cornea is gently indented with such a lens, a closed angle can be gently opened, allowing the observer to differentiate *appositional* closure where there are no synechia from *synechial* closure where synechia are present (Figure 3.4) [11].

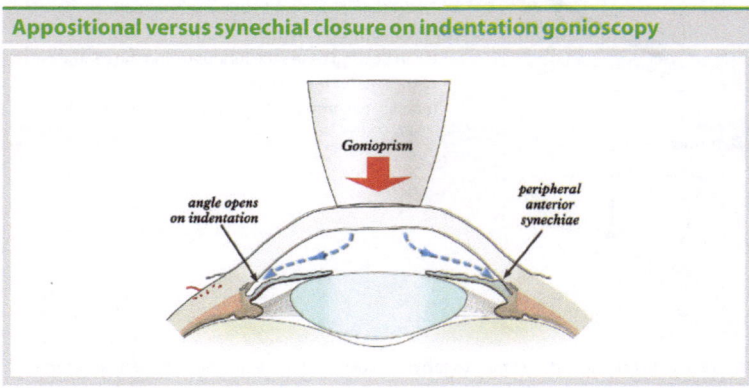

Appositional versus synechial closure on indentation gonioscopy

Figure 3.4 Appositional versus synechial closure on indentation gonioscopy. Courtesy of Alan Lacey , reproduced with permission from © Moorfields Eye Hospital, 2013. All Rights Reserved.

Angle grading systems

Angle depth is graded during gonioscopy (Figure 3.5) [12]. There are a number of systems for this (eg, the Shaffer, Spaeth, and Scheie systems); the Shaffer and Spaeth being the most well known. Table 3.1 shows the Shaffer system, which is the simplest [13]. The Spaeth system elaborates on this by grading the geometric angle between the cornea and iris, the peripheral iris contour and the position of the insertion of the iris root.

Comparison of normal anterior chamber angle and some examples of angle closure

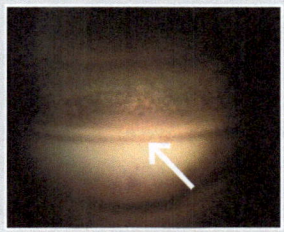

A wide open normal angle on gonioscopy. In this case there is some mild pigmentation of the trabecular meshwork (arrow)

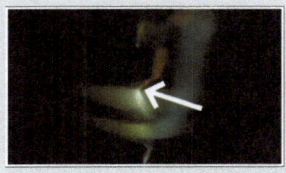

A closed angle on gonioscopy. It can sometimes be difficult to differentiate the appearance of a closed angle from an open angle with pale trabecular meshwork. In this case, the thin slit-beam section of the corneal wedge (the apex of the corneoscleral junction) indicates the position of Schwalbe's line (arrow). As the corneal wedge intersects at the iris root in this case, all normal iris structures are situated peripheral to the iris root, indicating that this angle is closed

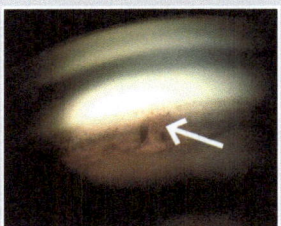

An isolated peripheral anterior synechia (arrow) attaching the peripheral iris to Schwalbe's line. This example is rather more dramatic than those typically seen in primary angle closure and is more characteristic of uveitic glaucoma

Figure 3.5 Comparison of normal anterior chamber angle and some examples of angle closure.

The Schaffer angle grading system

Grade	Angle depth (angle between posterior corneal wall and anterior iris face)
4	45°
3	>20° and <40°
2	20°
1	10°
Slit	<10°
0	Angle is closed

Table 3.1 The Schaffer angle grading system. This article was published in *The Glaucomas*, Second edition, Ritch et al, © Elsevier (1996). Adapted from the American Academy of Ophthalmology [13].

Other methods of imaging the iridocorneal angle

It is increasingly common to look for iridotrabecular contact in the eyes of patients with narrow angles that might be occludable, using anterior segment optical coherence tomography. This technique has the advantage that it does not involve instrument contact with the eye and also that it can be used to derive measurements of the anterior chamber angle in each quadrant of each eye in the light and in the dark. As mentioned above it has the disadvantage that specific abnormalities in the angle cannot be visualized.

Dilated fundus examination and optic disc evaluation

Dilated examination is essential not only to examine the optic disc in detail for signs of glaucomatous changes, but to exclude other posterior segment abnormalities that could results in secondary glaucoma, such as diabetic retinopathy, evidence of previous retinal detachment surgery and lens abnormalities, such as subluxation and exfoliation syndrome, as well as to look for signs of cataract.

The pupil is dilated to enable a stereoscopic view of the posterior segments of the eye. This method enables assessment of any characteristic glaucomatous signs, including cupping (excavation) at the optic disc, optic disc hemorrhages and retinal nerve fiber layer defects. The eye is anaesthetized when using a contact lens.

An assessment of the optic disc (Table 3.2) is fundamental to the diagnosis of glaucoma. Characteristic glaucomatous signs include cupping (excavation) and nerve loss at the optic disc (Figure 3.6) [14].

Factors to consider when evaluating the optic disc

Factor
Size of the optic disc
Size and shape of the excavation (cupping)
Vertical cup:disc ratio
Peripapillary atrophy (atrophy around the optic disc)
Visibility of and defects in the retinal nerve fiber layer

Table 3.2 Factors to consider when evaluating the optic disc.

Appearance of the optic disc in a healthy eye and a glaucomatous eye

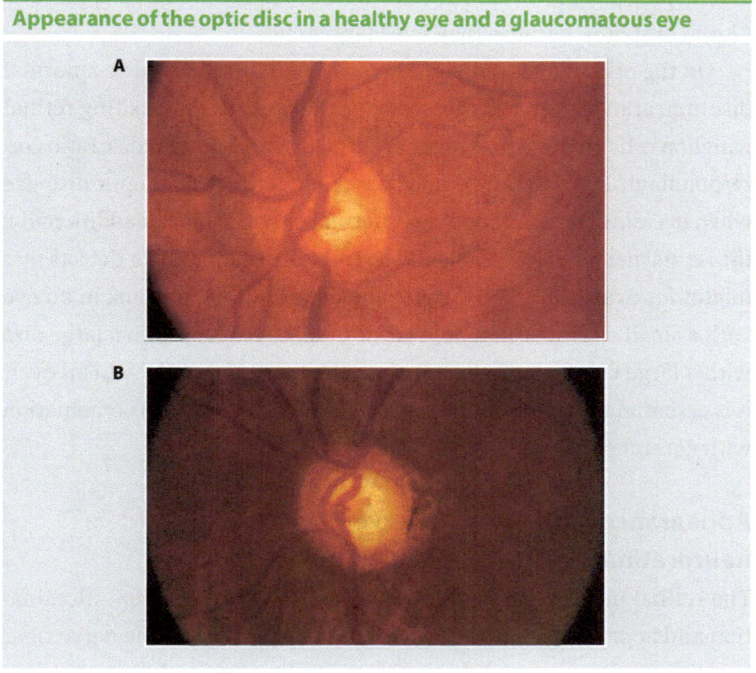

Figure 3.6 Appearance of the optic disc in a healthy eye and a glaucomatous eye. A, Normal cupping with healthy neuroretinal rim; **B**, the optic disc shows inferior and temporal thinning of the disc rim as well as baring of the supranasal artery, which are signs of glaucomatous damage. In addition, disc cupping can be generalized along the whole neuroretinal rim. Reproduced with permission from Fantes and Anderson [14].

Size of the optic disc

The size of the optic disc can be estimated by measuring the height of the slit beam, which is equal to the diameter of the optic disc as viewed through a condensing lens and slit lamp directly. A magnification correction factor is used to adjust for differing strengths of condensing lens. Modern imaging devices, such as scanning laser ophthalmoscopes, also measure optic disc size.

The number of optic nerve fibers is similar irrespective of the size of the disc, and is roughly 1.2 million. The normal optic disc is 1.5–2 mm in vertical diameter. Individuals with larger optic discs will have a larger cup:disc ratio than those with smaller discs. This can easily lead to a suspicion of glaucoma in patients who simply have large optic discs (2 mm or more), because they have larger cups.

On the other hand, individuals with small discs may have a normal disc appearance even with glaucoma; this is because the exiting retinal ganglion cells (RGC) axons are more crowded and the cup:disc ratio correspondingly less. For this reason it is essential to consider optic disc size when deciding whether cupping is normal or pathological; additionally, the retinal nerve fiber layer should be carefully examined for defects that might, for example, add weight to the diagnosis of glaucoma in an eye with a small optic disc that appears normal, or reassure that a large disc with a large cup:disc ratio is not glaucomatous (Figure 3.7). In all eyes, it is essential that these structural assessments be made in combination with careful examination of the visual field.

Appearance of the retinal nerve fiber layer and neuroretinal rim

The retinal nerve fiber layer is viewed with red-free (green) illumination and appears as fine, silvery striations, representing the nerve fiber bundles. The presence of defects strongly suggests pathology because less than 3% of normal eyes demonstrate them. With gradual loss of nerve fibers over time, the layer thins and becomes harder to see as glaucoma progresses (Figure 3.8A). Focal defects are easier to detect than generalized thinning.

Appearance of a small-, medium- and large-sized normal optic discs with varying degrees of physiological excavation

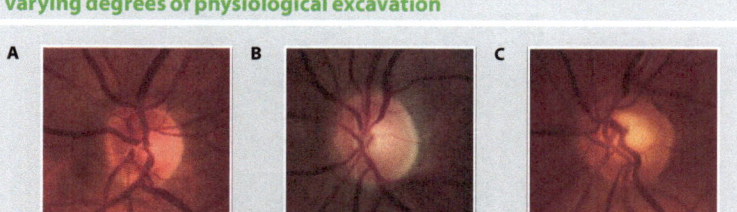

Figure 3.7 Appearance of a small-, medium- and large-sized normal optic discs with varying degrees of physiological excavation. The optic disc on the left is rather small (approximately 1.5 mm vertical diameter) and consequently less cupped than that in the middle (1.7 mm vertical diameter). The disc on the right is larger (2.0 mm vertical diameter) and more cupped, even though this is also a normal optic disc. It is important in such cases to examine the retinal nerve fiber layer to distinguish normality from abnormality. These images are not corrected for magnification. Reproduced with permission from © David Garway-Heath, 2013 [15]. All Rights Reserved.

It is important when examining for nerve fiber layer defects to use a relatively low magnification. Often a 90D lens gives a better view of the posterior pole for this purpose than many of the more specialized modern lenses. Retinal nerve fiber layer (splinter) hemorrhages (Figure 3.8B) may be seen in the neuroretinal rim of the optic disc in up to a third of glaucoma patients at some time in the course of the disease, as compared with less than 0.2% of the normal population. In general these are a sign that the patient's glaucoma is likely to be progressing. A number of imaging devices also give measurements of the retinal nerve fiber layer, which may assist in evaluation. These include scanning laser polarimetry (GDX, Carl Zeiss Meditec, Dublin, CA), confocal scanning laser ophthalmoscopy (Heidelberg Retinal Tomography, Heidelberg Engineering) and optical coherence tomography.

Shape of the excavation (cupping)

Usually the neuroretinal rim is widest inferiorly, then superiorly, nasal and temporally in decreasing order of thickness (Figure 3.9). This has led to the development of the "ISNT rule" by Jonas. In the absence of clear a developmental anomaly of the optic disc, failure to follow the *ISNT* rule is suggestive, but not diagnostic of glaucomatous optic neuropathy.

Retinal nerve fiber layer defect

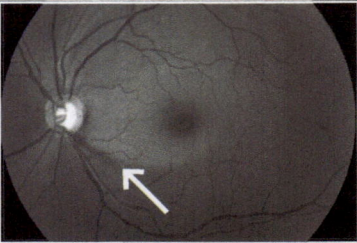

Figure 3.8A Retinal nerve fiber layer defect. This is rather obvious (arrow), and often the defect may be rather subtle. It is important and helpful to use lower magnification (eg, 90D lens) and use a red-free (green) filter. Reproduced with permission from © Moorfields Eye Hospital, 2013. All Rights Reserved.

Optic disc hemorrhage

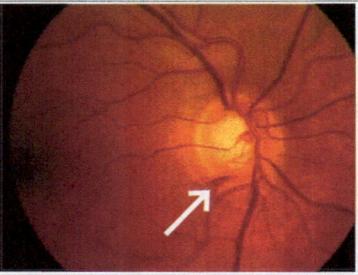

Figure 3.8B Optic disc hemorrhage. Reproduced with permission from © Moorfields Eye Hospital, 2013. All Rights Reserved.

Glaucomatous optic disc with significant loss of rim in all quadrants

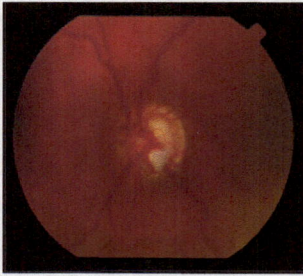

Figure 3.9 Glaucomatous optic disc with significant loss of rim in all quadrants. There is additionally a deep notch in the inferior pole of the disc. Reproduced with permission from © Moorfields Eye Hospital, 2013. All Rights Reserved.

Asymmetry of the optic disc cups between the two eyes may also be due to a congenital anomaly and it is important to measure the disc size on slit-lamp examination as asymmetry of cup:disc ratio sometimes simply reflects asymmetry in vertical disc diameter. If both discs exhibit no signs of a congenital anomaly and are similar in vertical diameter, then evidence of cup asymmetry is suggestive of glaucomatous change.

Vertical cup:disc ratio

The vertical cup:disc ratio has long been used in the assessment of the glaucoma suspect. A large cup:disc ratio is suggestive of glaucoma or other pathology; however, the wide range of values for this ratio in the normal population limits its use (Figure 3.10) [10]. In a large normal disc, the cup:disc ratio is large and falsely suggests glaucoma.

Peripapillary atrophy

Peripapillary atrophy is characterized by the loss of retinal tissue, exposing the underlying sclera (Figure 3.11). Its location may correlate with that of visual field defects. A temporal crescent of peripapillary atrophy is common in normal eyes. Thus, it is not diagnostic of glaucoma; however,

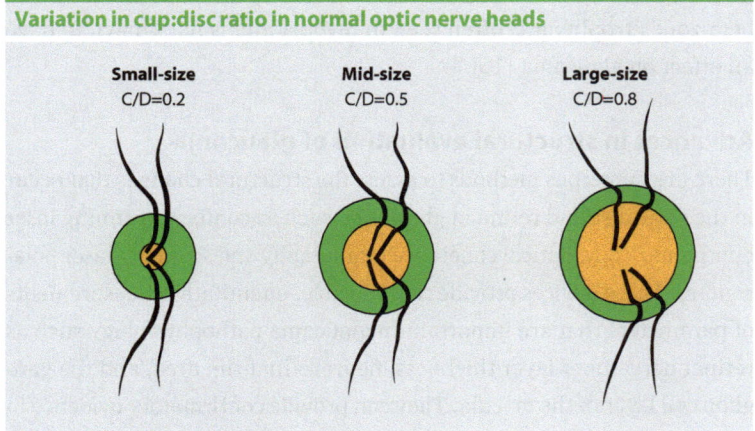

Figure 3.10 Variation in cup:disc ratio in normal optic nerve heads. Optic nerve heads with different disc area but with the same rim area and same retinal fiber number: small-size disc (disc area <2 mm² and C/D=0.2); mid-size disc (disc area between 2 and 3 mm² and C/D=0.5); and large-disc (disc area >3 mm² and C/D=0.8). C/D, cup:disc ratio. Reproduced with permission from © European Glaucoma Society, 2013 [10]. All Rights Reserved.

Signs of glaucomatous peripapillary atrophy

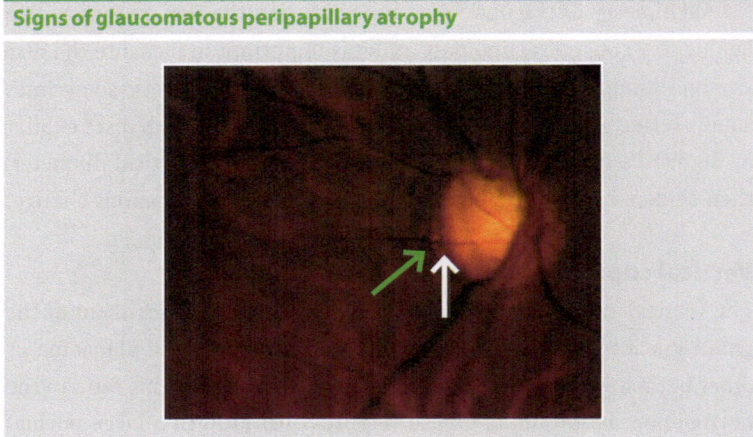

Figure 3.11 Signs of glaucomatous peripapillary atrophy. Reproduced with permission from © Moorfields Eye Hospital, 2013. All Rights Reserved.

any increase in the extent of the atrophy indicates a disease process, such as glaucoma or progressive myopia, thus is should be regarded as an extra clue that glaucoma may be present.

There are two types of peripapillary atrophy. Beta-zone atrophy occurs adjacent to the optic disc and is more frequent and extensive in glaucoma than in normal eyes. Alpha-zone atrophy occurs peripheral to beta-zone atrophy; it is often seen in myopia and is not known to have an effect on glaucoma [16].

Advances in structural evaluation of glaucoma

There are numerous methods to assess the structural changes that occur in the optic disc and retina in glaucoma, such as confocal scanning laser ophthalmoscopy, optical coherence tomography and scanning laser polarimetry. These devices provide reproducible, quantitative measurements of parameters that are important in glaucoma pathophysiology such as retinal nerve fiber layer thickness, neuroretinal rim area, and the ganglion cell layer of the macula. They can provide confirmatory evidence in glaucoma diagnosis and progression when evaluated in conjunction with the appearance of the optic nerve and visual field but are not suitable for use as stand-alone diagnostic tools or screening devices.

Automated perimetry

Automated perimetry is essential in making the diagnosis of glaucoma, monitoring disease progression and assessing the efficacy of therapy. Visual field abnormalities may also occur in association with congenital anomalies of the optic nerve, and also with cerebrovascular disease. In general, regular evaluation over time will help to differentiate a visual field defect due to glaucoma (ie, the case is usually progressive if untreated or inadequately treated) from one due to a developmental abnormality or a stroke (ie, the defect should be stationary). Obviously there are other causes of visual field defects and other features of cerebrovascular disease that would suggest the diagnosis; however, it is essential to perform a baseline visual field examination when a patient first presents so that further change can be detected.

Several systems are available. The two most common systems are the Humphrey® Field Analyzer and the Octopus Perimeter™. Ideally, a patient should be monitored over time using the same type of machine and same testing algorithm on each occasion so that sequential field test results are comparable.

Figure 3.12 shows examples of moderate and severe visual field defects. There are many systems for staging functional damage in glaucoma, according to classification of visual field defects; however, a recent review of systems for staging severity and for distinguishing types of field loss over the last 40 years concluded that none of the systems are in widespread clinical use [17].

Investigating ocular perfusion

In patients, especially those with normal-pressure glaucoma or Raynaud's phenomenon, it may be appropriate to investigate the possibility of reduced perfusion. In such cases, 24-hour systemic blood pressure measurement may be of value. Patients with well-controlled IOP who demonstrate progressive worsening of glaucoma are sometimes found to have nocturnal systemic hypotension. This is believed to be especially true of those who are treated aggressively for systemic hypertension and occasionally it is

Visual field defects in glaucomatous patients

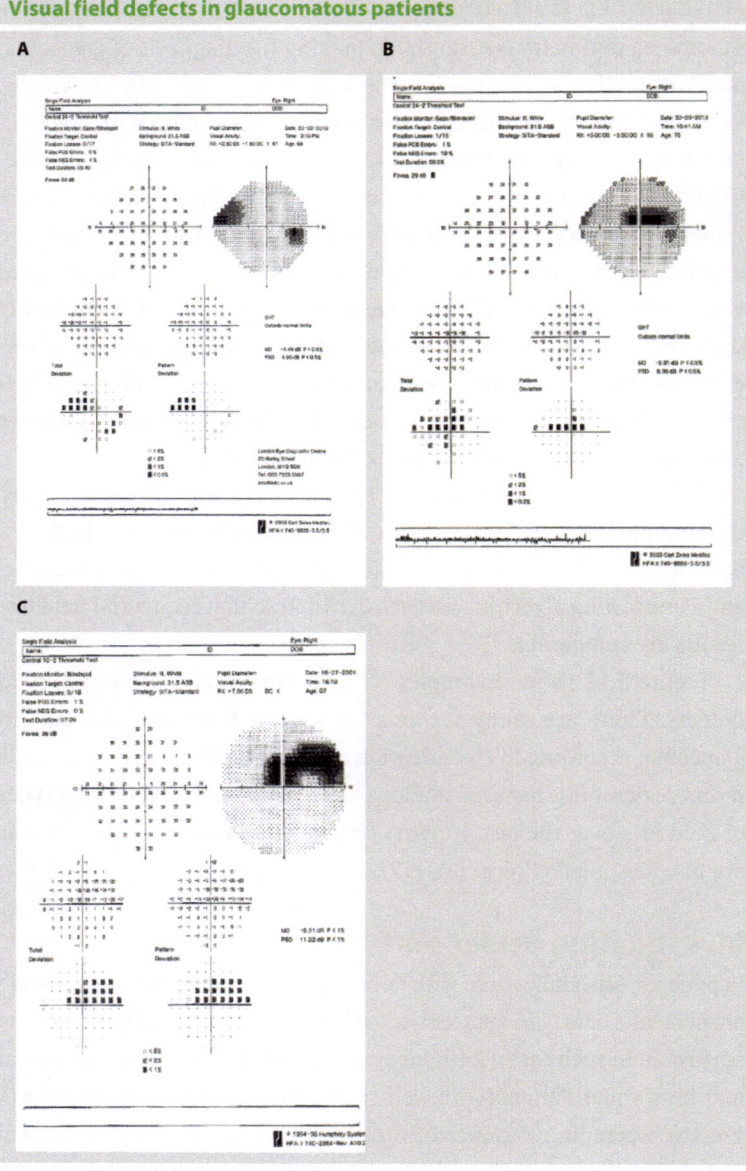

Figure 3.12 Visual field defects in glaucomatous patients. A, right nasal step seen in using the Humphrey Field Analyzer II and the 24-2 SITA standard algorithm; **B,** right upper arcuate scotoma seen on 24-2 SITA standard threshold perimetry; **C,** the same right upper arcuate scotoma on a different date using the 10-2 algorithm to visualize the central 10 degrees only. Reproduced with permission from © Moorfields Eye Hospital, 2013. All Rights Reserved.

useful to review the patient's systemic antihypertensive medication in collaboration with their general physician.

Conclusions

The most important signs of glaucomatous optic nerve damage are a characteristic structural change in the optic disc and retinal nerve fiber layer, and a progressive visual field loss. It is important to correlate visual field changes with optic disc changes when possible. A patient who presents with both visual field and optic disc changes that are characteristic of glaucoma, with or without family history of glaucoma and with or without elevated IOP, will require careful management to prevent further glaucomatous damage and worsening of visual field.

References

1   Doughty MJ, Zaman ML. Human corneal thickness and its impact on intraocular pressure measures: a review and meta-analysis approach. *Surv Ophthalmol.* 2000;44:367-408.

2   Brandt JD, Beiser JA, Kass MA, et al. Central corneal thickness in the Ocular Hypertension Treatment Study (OHTS). *Ophthalmology.* 2001;108:1779-1788.

3   Leske MC, Heijl A, Hyman L, et al. EMGT Group. Predictors of long-term progression in the early manifest glaucoma trial. *Ophthalmology.* 2007;114:1965-1972.

4   van Herick W, Shaffer RN, Schwartz A. Estimation of width of angle of anterior chamber: Incidence and significance of the narrow angle. *Am J Ophthalmol.* 1969;68:626-629.

5   Foster PJ, Devereux JG, Alsbirk PH, et al. Detection of gonioscopically occludable angles and primary angle-closure glaucoma by estimation of limbal chamber depth in asians: modified grading scheme. *Br J Ophthalmol.* 2000;84:186-192.

6   Drance SM. The significance of the diurnal tension variations in normal and glaucomatous eyes. *Arch Ophthalmol.* 1960;64:494-501.

7   Barkana Y, Anis S, Liebmann J, et al. Clinical utility of intraocular pressure monitoring outside of normal office hours in patients with glaucoma. *Arch Ophthalmol.* 2006;124:793-797.

8   Hughes E, Spry P, Diamond J. 24-hour monitoring of intraocular pressure in glaucoma management: a retrospective review. *J Glaucoma.* 2003;12:232-236.

9   Foster PJ, Aung T, Nolan WP, et al. Defining "occludable" angles in population surveys: drainage angle width, peripheral anterior synechia, and glaucomatous optic neuropathy in east Asian people. *Br J Ophthalmol.* 2004;88:486-490.

10 European Glaucoma Society. *Terminology and Guidelines for Glaucoma.* 3rd edition. Savona, Italy: Dogma; 2008.

11 Cyrlin MN. Primary and secondary angle-closure glaucomas. In: Schacknow PN, Samples JR, eds. *The Glaucoma Book: A Practical Evidence-Based Approach to Patient Care.* New York: Springer Science+Business Media, LLC, 2010.

12 Dawczynski J, Koenigsdoerffer E, Augsten R, Strobel J. Anterior optical coherence tomography: a non-contact technique for anterior chamber evaluation. *Graefe's Arch Clin Exp Ophthalmol.* 2007;245:423-425.

13 American Academy of Ophthalmology: The Eye M.D. Association. *2011-2012 Basic and Clinical Science Course, Section 10: Glaucoma.* San Francisco, CA: American Academy of Ophthalmology; 2011.

14 Fantes F, Anderson D. In: Parrish E II, Budenz DL, eds. *The University of Miami Bascom Palmer Eye Institute Atlas of Ophthalmology*. Philadelphia, PA: Current Medicine Group LLC; 2000.

15 Garway-Heath DF, Ruben ST, Viswanathan A, et al. Vertical cup/disc ratio in relation to optic disc size: its value in the assessment of the glaucoma suspect. *Ophthalmology*. 1998;82:1118-1124.

16 Jonas JB, Budde WM, Panda-Jonas S. Ophthalmoscopic evaluation of the optic nerve head. *Surv Ophthalmol*. 1999;43:293-320.

17 Brusini P, Johnson CA. Staging functional damage in glaucoma: review of different classification methods. *Surv Ophthalmol*. 2007;52:156-179.

Chapter 4

Medical management of glaucoma

Overview

Treatment of glaucoma is long term; thus, it needs to be supplemented by a holistic approach to the patient, including education about the condition and the aim of treatment, support with continuing therapy, including instillation of medication, and measures to improve general health. Management has to be tailored to the individual needs of each patient to maximize the efficacy of treatment in maintaining visual function and related quality of life. The treatment options currently available are:

- medical therapy (usually in the form of eye drops);
- laser therapy (primarily trabeculoplasty); and
- surgery (eg, trabeculectomy, nonpenetrating procedures or aqueous shunt implantation).

Medical therapy is the standard first-line treatment. The only licensed drugs are those that aim to prevent progression of glaucomatous damage by lowering intraocular pressure (IOP). Pharmacotherapy can be continued in the long-term provided it effectively reduces IOP, is well tolerated and there are no signs of progression of glaucomatous damage.

Laser therapy (argon laser trabeculoplasty or selective laser trabeculoplasty) may also be used as first-line therapy. In general, these treatments do not avoid the need for medical therapy and, therefore, are not often used as first-line treatment. Laser trabeculoplasty is often most useful in patients with mild IOP elevation who are intolerant of or nonadherent to medical regimens. Laser iridotomy is a mainstay of prevention and

K. Barton and R. A. Hitchings, *Medical Management of Glaucoma*,
DOI: 10.1007/978-1-907673-44-3_4, © Springer Healthcare 2013

treatment of angle closure. Laser iridotomy acts by relieving pupillary block (ie, the main precipitating cause of angle closure in predisposed eyes). Surgery is considered for patients in whom IOP is not sufficiently controlled with medical therapy; in those with progressive glaucomatous damage despite relatively good IOP control; in those who are intolerant of medication; unable to instill medication and in those who have advanced glaucoma damage at the time of presentation.

Figure 4.1 and Figure 4.2 show treatment stepladders for common forms of open-angle glaucoma, progressing through medical and treatment approaches [1,2]. Laser therapy and surgery are beyond the scope of this book and will not be discussed further. Instead, this chapter will concentrate on the principles of medical management of glaucoma, including important related issues, such as compliance and side effects.

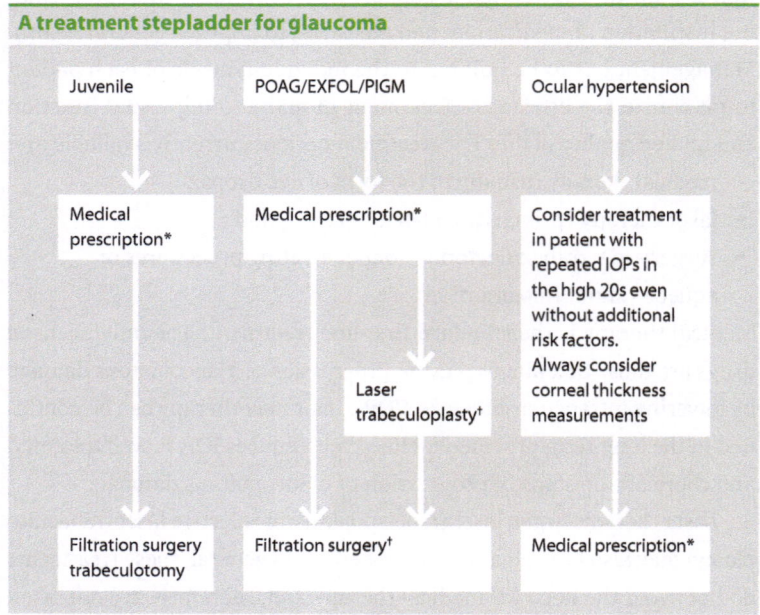

Figure 4.1 A treatment stepladder for glaucoma. If the above is not successful, consider repeat filtration surgery plus antimetabolites or aqueous drainage implant/cyclo destructive procedure. *Up to 2–3 different drugs (do not add a drug to a noneffective one; consider switching); †in certain cases, it may be necessary to consider filtration surgery without resorting to laser trabeculoplasty. EXFOL, exfoliative glaucoma; IOP, intraocular pressure; PIGM, pigmentary glaucoma; POAG, primary open-angle glaucoma. Reproduced with permission from © European Glaucoma Society, 2013 [1]. All Rights Reserved.

Treatment algorithm from the American Academy of Ophthalmologists Preferred Practice Pattern for primary open-angle glaucoma

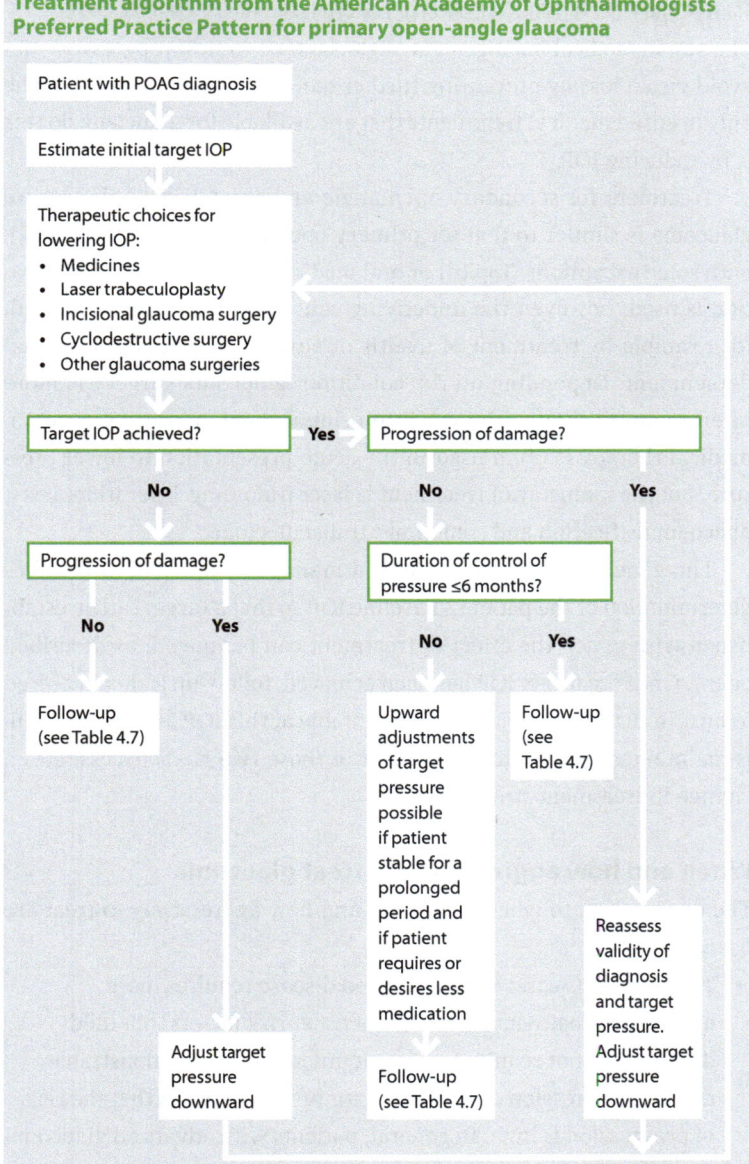

Figure 4.2 Treatment algorithm from the American Academy of Ophthalmologists Preferred Practice Pattern for primary open-angle glaucoma. IOP, intraocular pressure; POAG, primary open-angle glaucoma. Reproduced, with permission, from American Academy of Ophthalmology Glaucoma Panel. Preferred Practice Pattern® Guidelines. Primary Open-angle glaucoma. San Francisco, CA: © American Academy of Ophthalmology; 2010. Available at: www.aao.org/ppp [2].

Principles of medical management of glaucoma

The aim in medical management of glaucoma is to slow progression and avoid visual loss by preventing further damage to the optic nerve. The only licensed medical treatments that are available for glaucoma do this is by reducing IOP.

Treatment for secondary open angle and secondary angle-closure glaucoma is similar to that for primary open-angle glaucoma (POAG), with some exceptions. Topical or oral medication IOP-lowering medication is used; however, the underlying cause also has to be addressed, for example by treatment of uveitis or surgical correction of retinal detachment. Depending on the condition, glaucoma surgery is more often required than with POAG. In primary angle-closure glaucoma, medical therapy is often used in the acute presentation to lower pressure, but the mainstay of treatment is laser iridotomy, laser iridoplasty, phacoemulsification and sometimes trabeculectomy.

The general approach to medical management of POAG involves determination of the patient's baseline IOP so that a target can be established with which the effect of treatment can be judged, as described below. Once the target IOP has been achieved, follow-up is then required to ensure that the condition remains stable at this IOP and that the IOP is maintained. Failure to meet either of those two goals necessitates a change in treatment strategy.

When and how aggressively to treat glaucoma

The decisions as to whether to treat and how aggressively to treat are based on:

- *The stage of disease*: More advanced disease requires more aggressive treatment regardless of other risk factors, but mild disease may not require treatment unless there is demonstrable disease progression or the risk factor profile suggests that the risk of progression is high. In general, patients with advanced glaucoma at presentation should be considered as potential candidates for surgery. In particular, any patient with an advanced visual field defect or a visual field defect close to fixation at presentation are at a high risk of further visual loss and while it is normal to start with medical therapy, the above findings should be a warning sign that early surgery may be required.

- *The rate of progression,* as demonstrated by perimetry: The more rapid the rate of disease progression, the more likely it is that a patient will experience significant visual impairment for part of their life (Figure 4.3) [1]. It is important also to use common sense when advising treatment. In some patients, especially if they are particularly elderly and have a very slow rate of deterioration, aggressive treatment may be logistically difficult. The patient may not be able to put in their eye drops easily or may be forgetful. As with all aspects of treatment, but especially in this situation, it is important to discuss the risks and benefits of treating or not treating fully with the patient and any caregivers.

- *The life expectancy* of the patient: Caution is required in applying this in practice because life expectancy can be difficult to predict in older patients. As discussed above, in the situation where glaucomatous damage at diagnosis is not severe and progression is slow, the chances of significant visual impairment need to be

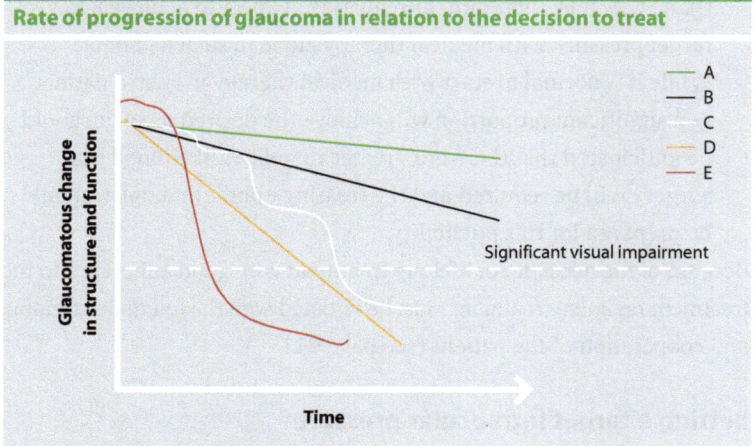

Figure 4.3 Rate of progression of glaucoma in relation to the decision to treat. The rate of glaucomatous damage varies between patients (eg, patients B to E) and can vary over time (eg, patients C and E). In normal eyes (patient A), normal age-related deterioration is too slow for significant impairment to occur within a normal lifespan. In patients with very slow deterioration, like patient B, deterioration may be too slow to warrant treatment. Patients C, D and E will require treatment. Reproduced with permission from © European Glaucoma Society, 2013 [1]. All Rights Reserved.

weighed against the disadvantages of treatment in the elderly. However, in younger patients (40–50 years of age), even slow progression could cause visual disability in their lifetime. This means a lower target pressure and closer visual field monitoring.

- *The degree of IOP elevation*: It is important to understand that IOP-lowering monotherapy can usually achieve a pressure drop of up to 35%. Combination therapy with multiple drugs may achieve a drop of up to 50%. Although it is common practice to use multiple drugs in patients who are not well-controlled, there is no evidence that using more than 2 to 3 drugs achieves additional pressure lowering. Worse still, the use of more than two "drop bottles" will reduce adherence to the treatment regime.

- If a patient presents with an untreated IOP level that is more than double the estimated target pressure then the likelihood that this will be achieved with medical therapy alone is less than 50%. For example, if a patient presents with advanced glaucoma and an untreated IOP level of greater than 30 mmHg, then the chance of achieving adequate IOP lowering with medical therapy is less than 50%. It is, therefore, unrealistic to expect to achieve a low target pressure with medical therapy alone in such a patient. While it is normal to start with medical therapy in such a patient as a significant proportion will achieve the desired level, it should be anticipated that there is a greater than 50% likelihood that surgery will be required and the treating ophthalmologist, should be prepared for this possibility.

Because of the necessity of lifelong treatment with good adherence to the treatment regimen, treatment must be initiated with the full understanding and cooperation of the patient (see page 91).

Setting a target intraocular pressure

Target IOP is the pressure at which damage is least likely to occur or progress. It varies between patients and can be different for each eye. It depends partly on the pre-treatment pressure; the lower the IOP at which damage has occurred, the lower the required target pressure. An extreme example of this is that the target pressure for normal-tension glaucoma (NTG) will be lower than that for high-tension glaucoma. The target IOP also depends how many additional risk factors for progression of glaucoma are present. Other factors that influence target IOP include those listed above for making the initial decision to treat glaucoma (ie, stage of disease, rate of progression, age and life expectancy) (see Figure 4.4) [1]. The presence of pseudoexfoliation is an independent risk factor for glaucoma progression [3].

Some authorities have set general targets. In the USA, for POAG the American Academy of Ophthalmology (AAO) recommends at least 20% below pre-treatment IOP [2]. In general, targets of less than 18 mmHg and less than 15 mmHg are often used. Lower targets are used for patients with more advanced glaucoma. The evidence base for these comes largely for the Advanced Glaucoma Intervention Study [4], but seems to be supported by subsequent trials, such as the Early Manifest Glaucoma Trial, which achieved a 25% reduction in IOP, medical therapy reduced the risk of glaucoma progression to 45%, compared with 62% for untreated controls [5].

The use of an exact target is controversial as the correct target cannot be identified in an individual patient with any precision and may need to be revised if insufficiently low and further progression occurs. One also

Factors that influence the setting of target intraocular pressure

Higher target IOP			
Early	Short	High	Slow
Glaucoma damage	**Life expectancy**	**Untreated IOP**	**Rate of progression**
Advanced	Long	Low	Fast
Lower target IOP			

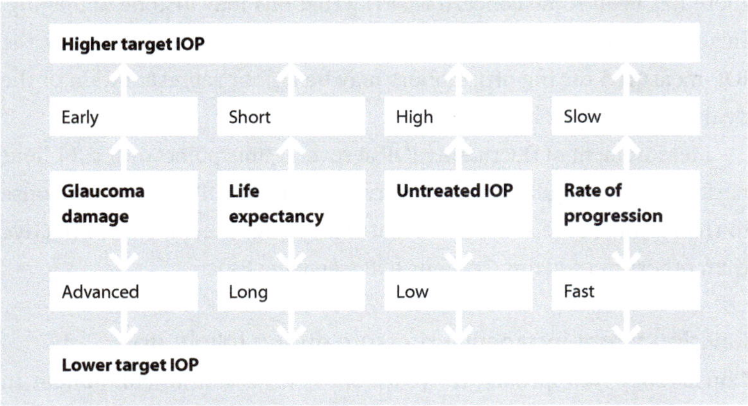

Figure 4.4 Factors that influence the setting of target intraocular pressure. The above factors need to be considered as a whole in deciding the individual target pressure required. IOP, intraocular pressure. Reproduced with permission from © European Glaucoma Society, 2013 [1]. All Rights Reserved.

runs the risk of setting unachievable targets. The target can only be judged to have been satisfactory after a period of stability of the visual field.

From a practical point of view, the target also needs to be relatively realistic. Most glaucoma specialists would agree that setting a target IOP level of, for example, 12 mmHg would be unnecessary and unrealistic for most patients, but might well be important in some situations (eg, a 40-years-old patient with advanced glaucoma at presentation or with a visual field defect threatening central fixation).

Diagnosing progression

Progression of glaucoma is normally diagnosed by observing a change in the visual field (Figure 4.5). It is important to be aware that visual field appearance may fluctuate quite significantly from one out-patient visit to the next. It is, therefore, important not to diagnose progression on two visual field test results alone and also to be aware that because of fluctuation in performance it can be difficult to diagnose progression accurately without the aid of analysis software.

Achieving a stable intraocular pressure

Achieving a stable IOP may be as important as achieving a low IOP. Marked fluctuations in IOP are observed in glaucomatous eyes and there has been some concern that fluctuations may also be damaging. In general, the importance of fluctuation in IOP is to highlight that the IOP measured during office hours may be a poor representation of the peak IOP over a 24-hour period.

Measurement of fluctuating IOP at several time points over a 24-hour period may be required to gain a true picture of IOP levels in response to treatment. There is evidence that some drugs may be more effective than others in reducing 24-hour IOP (see page 89).

Revising target intraocular pressure during follow-up

Consistency in approach to treatment is an essential component in maintaining the confidence of the patient. One factor that often causes patients confusion and loss of confidence in the physician is the frequent changing of medications.

Target IOP is not a fixed value, but rather a range at which we estimate that the risk of progression will be low. It will sometimes need to be revised. In general, a downward revision of target pressure is something that is only performed in the light of demonstrated consistent visual field progression on repeat visual field testing.

Starting and adjusting treatment

Unless there is severe damage and the IOP is very high, it is advisable to delay initiation of treatment until all appropriate baseline data have been collected. For example, it is important to record untreated IOP on more than one occasion (and it is useful to do this at different times of day) in order to have an accurate estimate of the baseline level with which to judge the effect of treatment. In most patients presenting with untreated IOP levels in the low- to mid-20s, this does not expose the patient to serious risk; however, there will be situations (eg, a very high presenting IOP or very advanced damage at presentation) where it will be more sensible to initiate treatment at the first visit.

It has been common practice to use a therapeutic trial in one eye before treating both eyes. The rationale is that this facilitates assessment of the efficacy of the drug or the extent to which the patient experiences side effects, without having to guess the effect of diurnal variation of IOP. In general therapeutic trials in one eye are poor predictors of the effect in the other eye and are no longer widely recommended.

Management is most difficult when target IOP is almost achieved but slow progression of glaucomatous damage continues. These are the patients where it is important to be realistic about the long-term chance of stabilizing their visual field on medical therapy alone. It is usual in such patients to increase medical therapy in a stepwise fashion, as suggested by the European Glaucoma Society and the AAO [1,2]; however, there is little extra benefit to be gained in treating a patient with more than three classes of agent (as previously discussed). If a patient is inadequately controlled on three classes of medical therapy, surgery to lower the IOP should be considered.

Example of visual field progression

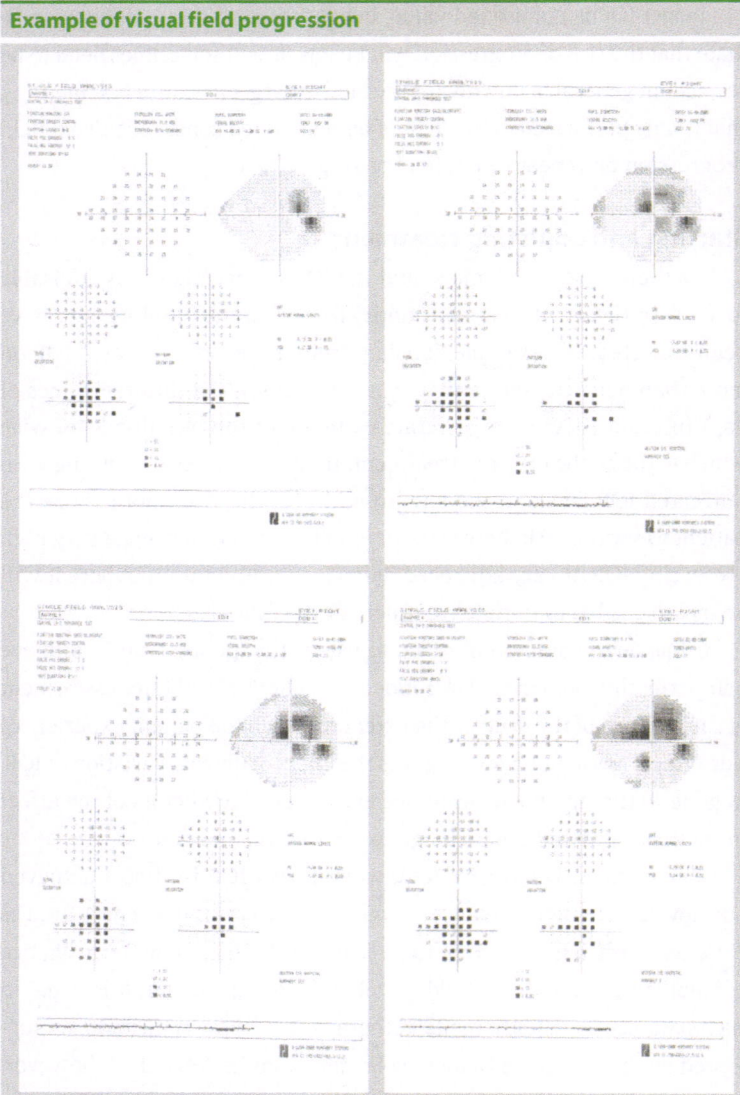

Figure 4.5 Example of visual field progression (continues opposite/overleaf).

Example of visual field progression (continued)

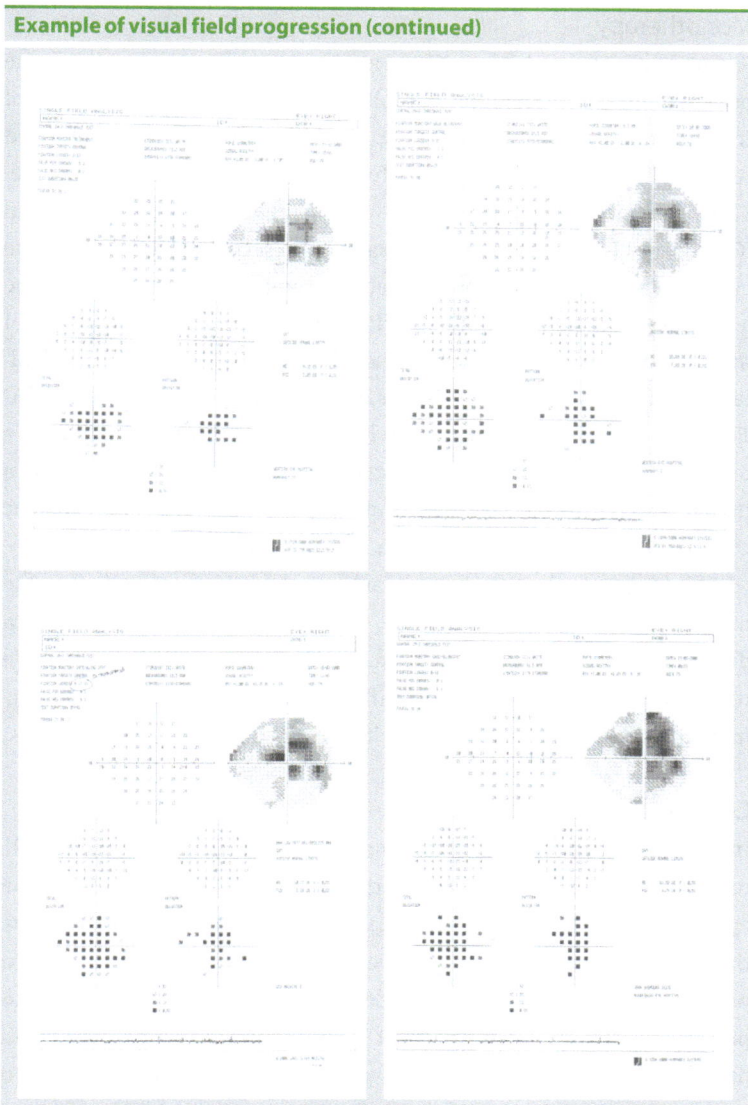

Figure 4.5 Example of visual field progression (continued). The visual field series shown here represents a consecutive series of eight 24–2 visual fields performed on one patient over a 4-year period, demonstrating clear evidence of visual field progression. In this patient, the visual field was eventually stabilized by trabeculectomy surgery with mitomycin C after which the IOP remained consistently below 12 mmHg. Prior to surgery, the IOP had been apparently well controlled at around 15 mmHg, during clinic attendances, but on diurnal measurement was found to peak at 18–20 mmHg. IOP, intraocular pressure. Reproduced with permission from © Moorfields Eye Hospital, 2013. All Rights Reserved.

Monotherapy

For most patients, medical treatment is a necessary inconvenience; in some patients, there are tolerability problems or a financial cost. The aim of treatment is, therefore, to use a regimen that can achieve the intended result with the fewest number of drop instillations that are practicable. Thus, treatment should be started with a single drug unless the initial IOP is very high, as it can be, for example, in secondary glaucoma. The current first-line options for the medical management of glaucoma are a topical prostaglandin analogue (PGA) or beta-blocker. The choice of drug depends on several factors, including the patient's age, concomitant disease and cost. In most cases, the usual first-line agent is a PGA. These produce slightly greater IOP lowering than beta-blockers with a once-daily dosage. For example, because most patients are elderly and a high proportion of elderly patients are already on treatment for cardiac conditions, beta-blockers may not a first-line choice.

If initial monotherapy does not achieve the IOP target, as is the case in more than 50% of patients [6,7], then either an additional drug or a different drug should be considered. If there has been no demonstrable response to the first drug, then clearly a different drug is indicated. It is more logical, in this situation to switch to a drug from a different class.

Combination therapy

In the above scenario, if a demonstrable response (ie, at least 20% reduction) in IOP has been achieved with the first drug, then it may be appropriate to add a second drug. Fixed combinations of two drugs have the theoretical advantage of improved adherence as the patient needs to put in fewer drops each day and experiences a lower overall exposure to preservatives; however, if IOP is not ideally controlled on a fixed combination of two drugs, sometimes it is worth splitting the combination into its individual components. While fixed combinations of beta-blockers and topical carbonic anhydrase inhibitors (CAI) seem to be equally efficacious as their individual components, there have been some concerns that fixed combinations of PGA and beta-blockers are slightly less efficacious than their individual components given separately; surprisingly, evidence to date shows little efficacy over PGA in isolation.

If a combination of two drugs (eg, PGA plus beta-blocker) is insufficient to control the IOP, it is useful to add a third drug (eg, a topical CAI). In that situation there is more evidence to support the use of a fixed combination of beta-blocker and topical CAI with a separate PGA than a fixed combination of beta-blocker and PGA with a separate topical CAI.

If this type of regimen is insufficient to control the IOP, there is little logic in adding a fourth drug, other than as a short-term holding strategy while awaiting surgery. There is a law of diminishing returns with increasing numbers of medications in that significantly better long-term IOP-lowering is unlikely, adherence diminishes, intolerance increases and for that reason a patient who is uncontrolled on three drugs should be offered surgery.

An alternative drug would be an alpha-agonist. In the authors' practices, these are often used in patients in whom beta-blockers are contraindicated, though they may also be considered as a third-line alternative to a topical CAI.

It should be remembered, however, that recent evidence suggests that topical preservatives can cause surface irritation in some eyes and, therefore, may reduce adherence.

When to treat ocular hypertension and normal-tension glaucoma

Ocular hypertension

Treating ocular hypertension (OHT) has benefits. For example, in the Ocular Hypertension Study of over 1600 patients with OHT, using medication to lower IOP achieved a reduction of 22.5%, almost half the risk of conversion to mild glaucoma during the 5-year study period [8]; however, the decision to treat patients with OHT is made on a case-by-case basis. It is worth pointing out that most of those converting in that particular study were diagnosed on changes in optic disc structural appearance before demonstrable visual field loss. As for patients with glaucomatous damage, IOP and the presence of additional risk factors are important considerations. Treatment should be initiated when the IOP is high enough to cause optic nerve damage or visual field loss.

The IOP level at which treatment should be initiated in OHT is still debated because the number needed to treat is high, as are the costs.

For example, a study to develop a model for estimating the global risk of disease progression in patients with OHT showed that in untreated patients the estimated risk of progression from OHT to unilateral blindness was 1.5–10.5% over 15 years [9]. In treated patients, the estimated risk of progression from OHT to unilateral blindness was 0.3–2.4% over 15 years. From these estimates, the number needed to treat to prevent one patient with OHT from progressing to unilateral blindness over a 15-year period was between 12 and 83. In a recent US study of cost-effectiveness of treating OHT [10], the authors concluded that it was not cost effective to treat all patients with OHT as the average incremental cost-effectiveness ratio was $89,072 per patient [10]; however, they suggested that treating selected patients with OHT and specific risk factors, such as advanced age, higher IOP and larger vertical cup:disc ratios, was cost-effective for preventing the onset of glaucomatous damage. Thresholds of 28–30 mmHg have been suggested; above these levels the likelihood of glaucomatous optic neuropathy (GON) becomes much higher if left untreated.

Treatment may be postponed for patients who are monitored regularly for changes in visual field and optic disc appearance. In reality, in developed countries, patients with OHT left untreated initially should not progress to blindness because they will be monitored and treatment will be initiated if signs of GON begin to develop. In contrast, the threshold for treatment should be lower in patients for whom regular monitoring will not possible.

Treatment of normal-tension glaucoma

Patients with evidence of GON and consistently normal IOP levels often progress more slowly than patients whose eyes have high IOP levels; however, NTG is also often diagnosed in the presence of more advanced disease (ie, the lack of a high IOP failing to alert the examiner during routine eye testing). While a proportion of patients with NTG do not deteriorate in the short-term, IOP-lowering treatment is required to prevent progression if it does occur. Similar to patients with elevated IOP, those who have advanced glaucoma at presentation or visual field defects close to fixation should be treated more aggressively to try to achieve low–normal IOP levels. While NTG patients may develop damage when the pressure is in the normal range, there is usually a history of mean pressures in the upper half of the normal range. In these patients a substantial reduction in IOP has been shown to be beneficial in terms of the course of disease in around 60% of patients with NTG [11].

However, in a significant minority of patients with NTG, visual field progression occurs despite IOP levels that appear to be consistently in the lower half of the normal range. In this category of patient, the treatment is still to lower IOP further in an attempt to achieve consistently low IOP levels around 10 mmHg. In those with systemic hypertension on treatment, it is also worth investigating the 24-hour systemic blood pressure profile.

Current therapeutic options for glaucoma

Pharmacotherapies for glaucoma reduce IOP by one of two mechanisms:

- reducing the production of aqueous humor (aqueous suppressants); and/or
- increasing the outflow of aqueous humor through the trabecular meshwork (conventional outflow) and/or the uveoscleral pathway.

Intraocular pressure-lowering drugs

Adrenergic agonists

Epinephrine, a nonselective adrenergic agent, was the first topical medication to be used in glaucoma almost a century ago and is now no longer used.

The alpha-2-selective agonists have been in use since the 1990s. These include apraclonidine and brimonidine. They are contraindicated in patients taking oral monoamine oxidase inhibitors (MAOI) antidepressants and infants. They act via both aqueous suppression and some increase in uveoscleral outflow, possibly via positive feedback on prostaglandin synthesis. They are generally used in 2–3 times daily dosing regimens and produce approximately 25% reduction in IOP levels. Tachyphylaxis may occur with these drugs and a significant proportion develops topical hypersensitivity reactions, periorbital lid injection, and ectropion and anterior uveitis in severe cases.

Beta-blockers

The beta-blockers have been used topically for glaucoma since the late 1960s and remain a useful class of drug for glaucoma therapy. They provide an effective alternative for initial monotherapy, are a popular choice for adjunctive therapy and are a component of many fixed-combination preparations because of their IOP-lowering efficacy both as monotherapy and as adjuncts. Beta-blockers are well-tolerated locally in the eye, but have significant respiratory and cardiovascular effects, reducing heart rate, and thereby blood pressure, and also causing bronchoconstriction. They are contraindicated in patients with respiratory disease, especially asthma, certain cardiovascular diseases and in frail, elderly patients [12].

Carbonic anhydrase inhibitors

Systemic CAIs have been used in the treatment of glaucoma for over 50 years and are an important therapeutic option in patients presenting acutely with very high IOP. Systemic symptoms and tachyphylaxis limit their long-term use and, in general, patients requiring systemic CAI are treated with these drugs only as an interim measure, either until any underlying cause of the IOP elevation is treated or until they have surgery to control the IOP [13].

Topical CAIs are generally used as second- or third-line to prostaglandins and beta-blockers. The topical medications and topical CAIs are described in Table 4.1 and oral CAIs in Table 4.2 [1,2].

Cholinergic agonists

Cholinergic agonists (miotics; parasympathomimetics) have been used in glaucoma therapy for over a century; however, because of their numerous side effects, they are often poorly tolerated and have been supplanted by newer medications during the past three decades. They are still useful in some individuals, primarily in the treatment of angle closure [14].

Prostaglandin derivatives

Prostaglandin derivatives have rapidly become the most commonly used ocular hypotensive agents since their introduction for glaucoma therapy in 1996, and are very effective first-line topical agents for lowering IOP [15].

The PGA have mostly replaced beta-adrenergic receptor antagonists as the treatment of choice for initial monotherapy. Patients can use contact lenses while using prostaglandin derivatives but should wait 15 minutes after administration before inserting the lenses.

Fixed-dose combinations of intraocular pressure-lowering drugs

A list of fixed-dose combination preparations is given in Table 4.3 [1]. Because all the fixed combinations contain a beta-blocker, contraindications to beta-blockers must be excluded.

Intraocular pressure-lowering drugs in pregnancy

If therapy is required during pregnancy, beta-blockers are usually used in isolation if possible as the cumulative experience with this class of drugs is greater than the more modern agents. Prostaglandin agonists should be avoided in pregnancy as these types of drug are used systemically to induce labor. There is less information with regard to the other drugs and these are best avoided. Glaucoma is relatively rare in women of child-bearing age and when it does occur it is often a secondary glaucoma, especially uveitic glaucoma. In these cases the IOP may be very high and occasionally surgery is required.

The role of preservatives in glaucoma drops

Concerns over the allergic and toxic effects of drop preservatives, particularly benzalkonium chloride, have resulted in the development of alternate preservatives and preservative-free topical medications. Brimonidine, an alpha-2 agonist, and travoprost, a prostaglandin derivative, have alternative preservative forms that benefit patients with benzalkonium allergy or toxicity, the latter affecting patients with ocular surface disease and tear film insufficiency. Timolol (beta-blocker), bimatoprost (PGA), latanoprost (PGA), tafluprost (prostaglandin derivative), and the fixed combination of timolol/dorzolamide are all available in preservative-free preparations.

Topical medical treatment for glaucoma: medications that reduce intraocular pressure

Drug class and mechanism of action	Drugs*	Major contraindications	Side effects
Selective alpha-2 adrenergic agonists: Decreases aqueous humor production (increases uveoscleral outflow: brimonidine)	Apraclonidine 0.5%, 1%; 2–3 times daily Brimonidine 0.15% 3 times daily or 0.2% twice daily	Infants and children aged 2 years and younger; previous allergy to alpha-agonists; monoamine oxidase inhibitor therapy	Dry mouth, eyelid elevation, allergy/hypersensitivity, local contact dermatitis, decreases systemic blood pressure, fatigue, somnolence, headache
Beta-blockers (beta-adrenergic receptor antagonists): Decreases aqueous humor production by the ciliary body by up to 50%	All given once or twice daily **Nonselective** • Carteolol 0.5–2% • Levobunolol 0.1–0.5% • Metipranolol 0.1–3% • Timolol 0.1–0.5%	**Nonselective:** asthma, history of obstructive pulmonary disease, sinus bradycardia, heart block, cardiac failure	**Nonselective:** systemic side effects include bradycardia, arrhythmia, heart failure, syncope, bronchospasm, airway obstruction, distal edema, hypotension, depression, masking of hypoglycemia in diabetes, nocturnal hypotension; ocular side effects include epithelial keratopathy, corneal sensitivity reduction
	Beta-selective: • Betaxolol 0.25–0.5%	**Beta-selective** (betaxolol): relative contraindication in same conditions	**Beta-selective** (betaxolol) better tolerated than nonselective but less effective at lowering the IOP
Carbonic anhydrase inhibitors (topical): Decreases aqueous humor production by inhibiting carbonic anhydrase in the ciliary body	• Dorzolamide 2%; twice daily • Brinzolamide 1%; twice daily	Hypersensitivity to product components	Burning, stinging, bitter taste, superficial punctuate keratitis, blurring, tearing, headache, urticaria, angioedema, pruritus, asthenia, dizziness, paresthesia, transient myopia, corneal edema

Table 4.1 Topical medical treatment for glaucoma: medications that reduce intraocular pressure (continues opposite/overleaf).

Topical medical treatment for glaucoma: medications that reduce intraocular pressure (continued)

Drug class and mechanism of action	Drugs*	Major contraindications	Side effects
Cholinergic agonists (parasympathomimetics)[†]: Increases trabecular meshwork	**Direct acting:** • Pilocarpine (0.5–4% eye drops 3 or 4 times daily; gel once daily)	**Direct acting:** Age <40 years, cataract, uveitis, neovascular glaucoma, worsening papillary block	**Ocular:** miosis, pseudomyopia, brow ache, retinal detachment, ciliary spasm, increased papillary block, decreased vision, cataract, periocular contact dermatitis, corneal toxicity **Systemic:** Intestinal cramp, bronchospasm
Prostaglandin analogues: Increases uveoscleral outflow of aqueous humor; bimatoprost also increases trabecular outflow	• Latanoprost 0.005%; once daily • Travoprost 0.004%; once daily • Bimatoprost 0.01% or 0.03%; once daily • Tafluprost 0.0015%; once daily	Hypersensitivity to any of the agents or ingredients, macular edema, history of herpetic keratitis	**Local/ocular:** conjunctival hyperemia, stinging, increase in periocular skin pigmentation and eyelash changes (both reversible), irreversibly increased iris pigmentation, reactivation of herpes keratitis, anterior uveitis, cystoid macular edema in aphakes/pseudoaphakes in some cases **Idiosyncratic:** dyspnea, asthma and asthmatic exacerbation

Table 4.1 Topical medical treatment for glaucoma: medications that reduce intraocular pressure (continued). *All preparations are eye drops unless otherwise stated; [†]The indirect-acting cholinergic agent acetylcholine is also used during surgery. IOP, intraocular pressure. Adapted from the European Glaucoma Society and the American Academy of Ophthalmology [1,2].

Systemic carbonic anhydrase inhibitors

Carbonic anhydrase inhibitors dosage	Major contraindications	Side effects	Wash out time
• Acetazolamide (tablets; 1000 mg/day: 250 mg tablet q.i.d. or 500 mg sustained release capsule b.i.d.) • Methazolamide (tablets; 50–100 mg/day: 25 mg or 50 mg; b.i.d. or t.i.d.)	Depressed sodium and/or potassium levels, kidney disease/ dysfunction, liver disease/dysfunction, suprarenal gland failure, hyperchloremic acidosis	Paresthesias, hearing dysfunction, tinnitus, appetite loss, taste alteration, gastrointestinal disturbances, depression, decreased libido, kidney stones, blood dyscrasias, metabolic acidosis, electrolyte imbalance, Stevens-Johnson syndrome, malaise, metallic taste in mouth	3 days

Table 4.2 Systemic carbonic anhydrase inhibitors. Adapted from the European Glaucoma Society and the American Academy of Ophthalmology [1,2].

Fixed-dose combination therapy for glaucoma

Bimatoprost (0.03%)–timolol (0.5%)

Brimonidine (0.2%)–timolol (0.5%)

Brinzolamide (1%)–timolol (0.5%)

Dorzolamide (2%)–timolol (0.5%)

Latanoprost (0.005%)–timolol (0.5%)

Pilocarpine (2%)–timolol (0.5%)

Pilocarpine (2%)–metipranolol (0.1%)

Pilocarpine (2%)–carteolol (2%)

Travoprost (0.004%)–timolol (0.5%)

Table 4.3 Fixed-dose combination therapy for glaucoma. Reproduced with permission from © European Glaucoma Society, 2013 [1]. All Rights Reserved.

Improving ocular perfusion

In patients where significant nocturnal systemic hypotension can be demonstrated it may be worth discussing the possibility of reducing systemic antihypertensive medication (in collaboration with the patient's general physician) or other methods of elevating the blood pressure at night. In patients with marked systemic hypertension and glaucoma, the opposite is probably true (ie, that the blood pressure should be adequately controlled) (Table 4.4) [16].

Some IOP-lowering drugs improve 24-hour ocular perfusion. These are discussed below.

Managing glaucoma for twenty-four hours

As discussed in Chapters 2 and 3, IOP elevation may vary over 24 hours and, in some patients, is more marked during the night. IOP-lowering agents have been shown to vary in their facility for the entire 24-hour period, and there is evidence that some may be more effective in this respect. For example, in a short-term study of previously untreated individuals with POAG, IOP was significantly decreased at all points by timolol, brimonidine, dorzolamide and latanoprost, but with different drugs there were differences in the intensity of the reduction at night (Figure 4.6) [17].

In the same study with dorzolamide and latanoprost the diastolic ocular perfusion pressure (DOPP) was significantly increased at all 24-hour time points compared with baseline. In contrast, timolol and brimonidine induced significant increases for only part of the 24-hour period and brimonidine was associated with reductions at some times and in mean 24-hour DOPP [17]. The authors concluded that 24-hour DOPP profiles should be investigated further, including in long-term use.

Improving adherence in patients with glaucoma

Poor adherence to ocular hypotensive therapy and delayed follow-up visits to monitor disease greatly contribute to failure of treatment to prevent progression in glaucoma patients. Patient education and good communication between the patient, ophthalmologist and other medical professionals is essential to achieve maximum benefit from treatment. It is essential that the patient uses their eye drops regularly and properly,

Treatment of reduced ocular perfusion	
Hypotension	**Strategies to treat hypotension:** • daily-light physical exercise; • ensure adequate fluid and salt intake; • cessation/substitution of medications that lower blood pressure as a side effect; • titration or schedule alteration for antihypertensive medications taken during the day for patients who experience night-time dips in blood pressure; • assessment for suitability of support stockings for patients with orthostatic hypotension; and • medications to increase blood pressure (eg, mineralocorticoids like fludrocortisone) are sometimes considered

Table 4.4 Treatment of reduced ocular perfusion. Adapted from Flammer [16].

Intraocular pressure levels over twenty-four hours in untreated and newly treated primary open-angle glaucoma

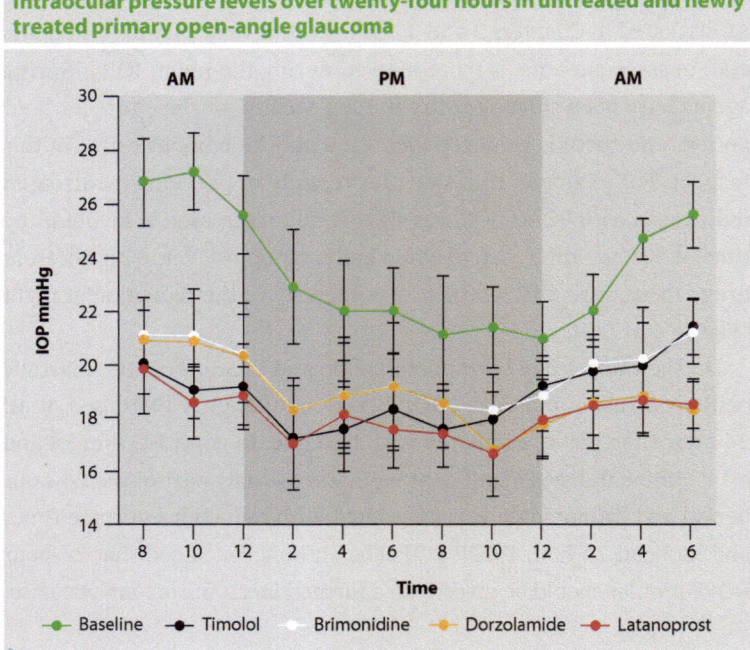

Figure 4.6 Intraocular pressure levels over twenty-four hours in untreated and newly treated primary open-angle glaucoma. IOP was measured at 2-hour intervals. IOP, intraocular pressure. Reproduced with permission from © Association for Research in Vision and Ophthalmology, Quaranta et al [17]. All Rights Reserved.

that they are instructed in how to instill them correctly, and that they understand the purpose and nature of treatment, including the reason for long-term treatment and monitoring. Methods that may improve adherence in patients with glaucoma are summarized in Table 4.5 and discussed in more detail below.

Providing information for the patient

Providing information about the disease and the methods of monitoring and treatment helps the patient understand the reason they have been prescribed the medication, and the importance of good adherence to the treatment regimen. Patients who adhere poorly to treatment are less likely to understand the link between glaucoma and blindness [18], and patients are more likely to adhere if they know the name of their eye disease [19].

Printed information for the patient to take away may be useful. It is also important to reiterate information about glaucoma and the rationale behind the treatment plan at return visits. The use of questionnaires to elicit information should also be considered; the patient may find it easier to report side effects or difficulties with compliance through a short questionnaire.

Ensuring medication is administered correctly

In a recent multicenter survey of Canadian glaucoma, patients found that more than 30% were administering their eye drops incorrectly: approximately 6% missed their eye completely and 28% contaminated the bottle [20]. Clearly, it is important to ensure that the patient, or the caregiver, knows how to instill the drops properly. In particular, they should be instructed on the need for sterile technique, the requirement that the eye is kept closed for at least a minute while drops take effect, drop separation time and how to reduce systemic absorption by pressing on the lacrimal duct. Patients who need more than one topical medication should be instructed to wait at least 5 minutes between instillations to avoid washout of the first drug.

Correct administration should be checked periodically at follow-up appointments. If IOP does not improve despite apparently adequate

Summary of methods to improve compliance in patients with glaucoma	
Dosing	• Tailor dosing times to daily events (eg, meals and bedtime)
Patient information	• Provide sufficient information about glaucoma and its treatment for the patient to understand the disease and the nature of treatment
Medication administration	• Ensure the patient or caregiver knows how to administer the eye drops properly
Treatment regimen	• Simplify the treatment regimen as much as possible • Keep any changes to the regimen simple • Consider using questionnaires to elicit information on difficulties with regimen • Avoid repetitive changes in treatment at consecutive visits
Side effects	• Explain possible side effects • Emphasize the importance of reporting any side effects experienced with treatment • Consider using questionnaires to elicit information
Patient monitoring	• Encourage the patient to have regular monitoring and explain that this is very important

Table 4.5 Summary of methods to improve compliance in patients with glaucoma.

therapy, it is worth asking the patient to demonstrate the administration method, so that feedback can be given if the method is faulty.

Simplifying the treatment regimen

Compliance decreases if administration of eye drops for glaucoma is more frequent than twice daily [21]. Patients are more likely to miss a dose if they are away from home in the middle of the day [22]. Compliance can be improved by prescribing daily dosing rather than twice daily dosing when possible, or using fixed combination therapy. Any changes to the treatment regimen should be kept simple, changing only one medication at a time. It is especially important to avoid repetitively treating medication at successive visits.

Tailoring dosing times to daily events, such as meals and bedtime, helps to cue the patient to take medications on schedule [22].

Explaining possible adverse effects

All medications used for the treatment of glaucoma may cause local and systemic adverse effects or induce an allergic reaction. Harmless, temporary effects, such as a slight burning sensation or eye redness, following topical administration are not an indication to discontinue treatment unless these effects are sufficient to adversely affect or reduce patient adherence, in which case another drug should be tried. If patients are forewarned, they may be more prepared to tolerate these milder adverse effects and may be more inclined to report their occurrence. On the other hand, more severe intolerance will require a change in medication. The decision to discontinue a medication in the presence of side effects is influenced not only by the severity of any reaction and the seriousness of the reaction, but also by the degree of IOP-lowering achieved in the individual patient by the drug in question and the likelihood of achieving a satisfactory IOP level with an alternative regimen.

It should be remembered that systemic side effects can also occur with topical eye preparations as they pass through the lacrimal duct and are absorbed through the nasal mucosa or throat. These are most often seen with beta-blockers with which systemic absorption is associated with a reversible reduction in peak flow in asthmatics and in the elderly.

Adverse effects related to preservatives

Some adverse effects, such as dry eye sensation, burning or stinging sensations, are due to benzalkonium chloride, the preservative used in most topical preparations [23]. Use of preservative-free preparations reduces these effects. For example, a study of over 4300 patients found a significant reduction ($P<0.001$) in adverse effects, such as discomfort upon instillation, and in symptoms between instillations, such as burning or stinging, foreign body sensation, dry eye sensation, tearing and eyelid itching [24]; however, there is a risk of infection with multiple-use bottles of preservative-free glaucoma medications: one study found that there was bacterial contamination of 8 out of 95 bottles collected from patients [25]. This problem can be circumvented by use of single-dose containers. At present, only one topical IOP-lowering therapy is available in this format: a dorzolamide–timolol combination supplied as a sealed sachet that contains 15 single-dose containers.

Monitoring the patient regularly

Patients should be encouraged to attend for regular monitoring and made aware that this ensures that any disease progression is observed as early as possible and allows treatment success to be judged. As well as providing an opportunity to check for tolerability and adherence.

Cost of glaucoma therapy

Treatment costs that are borne by the patient vary from country to country and are negatively correlated with efficacy largely due to reduced adherence [26,27].

Management of emergency situations

When IOP rises to extremely high levels, for example in acute primary angle-closure and in secondary glaucomas when it may rise to 50–80 mmHg, drugs to lower IOP are relatively ineffective as they cannot penetrate into the eye. Systemic IOP-lowering drugs are required in this situation, usually in advance of laser iridotomy or surgery. Acetazolamide is the most common drug used in this situation for acute IOP-elevation.

Acetazolamide can be administered intravenously or orally in doses of 500–1000 milligrams per day. Intravenous acetazolamide is very effective at lowering IOP in the first instance and is usually used in the emergency department to lower the IOP quickly. Ongoing treatment is usually with oral acetazolamide as a temporizing measure. Acetazolamide is not usually a good long-term treatment and patients who need acetazolamide for more than a few weeks will require surgery to control the IOP. It is also possible to treat children with intravenous acetazolamide (at reduced doses) in an emergency situation. If acetazolamide is insufficiently effective at reducing IOP in an emergency situation, hyperosmotic agents (oral glycerol or intravenous mannitol) can be used to further reduce the IOP. Mannitol has the advantage that it can be used effectively in patients who are vomiting, as is often the case with acute IOP elevation to high levels; however, mannitol can have a profound effect on the patient's fluid and electrolyte balance and should be used with caution in the elderly. Once the IOP is lowered sufficiently, topical drugs to reduce IOP can often be used to maintain IOP control.

Mechanisms to improve quality of life during treatment of glaucoma

Provided the patient does not have significant visual field loss or reduction in contrast sensitivity, and adheres to treatment and monitoring schedules, it should be possible to lead a normal or near-normal life. Approaches to optimizing quality of life are summarized in Table 4.6.

Follow-up

Once a target IOP level or range has been established and treatment instituted, follow-up is essential. It is important to ascertain whether the target level has been achieved or maintained, but more importantly to assess visual field or optic disc topographic status to ensure that the patient's glaucoma is stable. The European Glaucoma Society's recommendations for follow-up are shown in Figure 4.7 [1]; the AAO's recommendations for follow-up are shown in Table 4.7 [2]. IOP is tested at all follow-up visits. Visual fields will be performed at least annually and more often if there is a suspicion of change. The same is true of imaging tests. Gonioscopy should be repeated at each visit in patients with narrow angles.

Approaches to improving quality of life in patients with glaucoma	
Mechanism	**Effect**
Implement methods to maximize adherence	A patient who adheres to the treatment regimen and monitoring schedule is likely to benefit more from therapy than nonadherent patients and, therefore, gains quality of life benefits
Minimize disruption to the patient	Scheduling appointments and tests at times to suit the patient, when possible, encourages compliance with monitoring
Explain to the patient that some decrease in current quality of life (eg, inconvenience of treatment, reduced visual acuity following surgery) may ensure stabilization of future visual function	Patients who understand long-term goals of therapy may feel less demoralized by decrease in current quality of life
Ensure the patient's general practitioner is informed about the treatment regimen (directly and via the patient) because of possible systemic side effects	Drug interactions can be circumvented and contraindications can be considered
Consider fixed combination therapy if appropriate	Fixed combination therapy, rather than concomitant use of ≥2 drugs, simplifies treatment regimens and decreases inconvenience, which may improve quality of life
Address concerns commonly raised by patients	Advise patients that: • Coffee, tea and alcohol can be consumed in moderation • Regular physical exercise is encouraged; but sports, such as scuba diving, flying or extreme sports, should be discussed with the ophthalmologist • Playing of wind instruments should be discussed with the ophthalmologist. • Saunas can be used • Contact lenses can usually be worn after consulting the ophthalmologist

Table 4.6 Approaches to improving quality of life in patients with glaucoma.

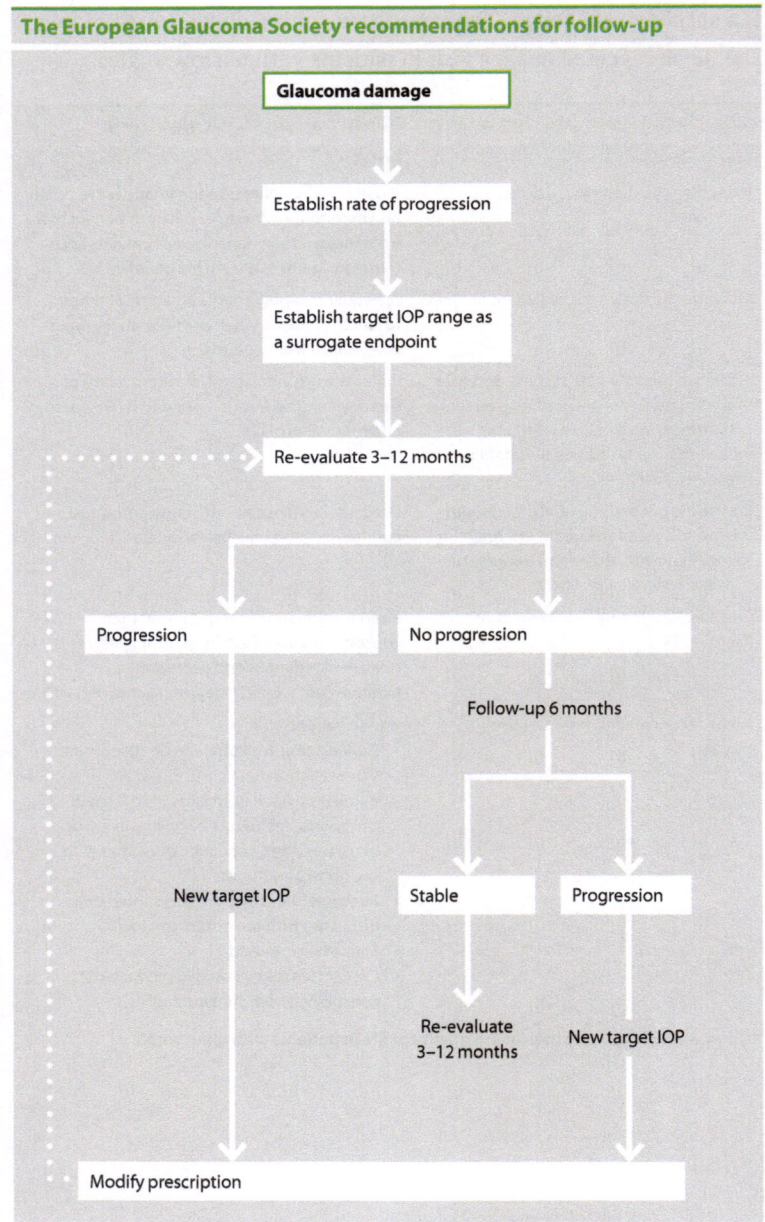

Figure 4.7 The European Glaucoma Society recommendations for follow-up. Follow-up intervals are just recommendations. IOP, intraocular pressure. Reproduced with permission from © European Glaucoma Society, 2013 [1]. All Rights Reserved.

American Academy of Ophthalmology recommendations for follow-up (glaucoma status evaluations with optic nerve and visual field assessment)

Target IOP achieved	Progression of damage	Duration of control (months)	Approximate follow-up interval (months)*
Yes	No	≤6	6
Yes	No	>6	12
Yes	Yes	NA	1–2
No	Yes	NA	1–2
No	No	NA	3–6

Table 4.7 American Academy of Ophthalmology recommendations for follow-up (glaucoma status evaluations with optic nerve and visual field assessment). Evaluations consist of clinical examination of the patient, include optic nerve head assessment (with periodic color stereophotography or computerized imaging of the optic nerve and retinal nerve fiber layer structure) and visual field assessment. *Patients with more advanced damage or greater lifetime risk from POAG may require more frequent evaluations. These intervals are the maximum recommended time between evaluations. IOP, intraocular pressure; NA, not applicable; POAG, primary open-angle glaucoma. Reproduced, with permission, from American Academy of Ophthalmology Glaucoma Panel. Preferred Practice Pattern® Guidelines. Primary Open-angle glaucoma. San Francisco, CA: © American Academy of Ophthalmology; 2010. Available at: www.aao.org/ppp [2].

References

1   European Glaucoma Society. *Terminology and Guidelines for Glaucoma*. 3rd edition. Savona, Italy: Dogma; 2008.

2   American Academy of Ophthalmology. Preferred practice pattern for primary open-angle glaucoma. San Francisco, CA: American Academy of Ophthalmology; 2010. Available at one. aao.org/asset.axd?id=56c908e3-a939-45ea-b12b-8fe609f547b0. Accessed August 7, 2013.

3   Leske MC, Heijl A, Hussein M, Bengtsson B, Hyman L, Komaroff E; Early Manifest Glaucoma Trial Group. Factors for glaucoma progression and the effect of treatment: the early manifest glaucoma trial. *Arch Ophthalmol*. 2003;121:48-56.

4   Primary open-angle. The Advanced Glaucoma Intervention Study (AGIS): 7. The relationship between control of intraocular pressure and visual field deterioration. The AGIS Investigators. *Am J Ophthalmol*. 2000;130:429-440.

5   Heijl A, Leske MC, Bengtsson B, et al; Early Manifest Glaucoma Trial Group. Reduction of intraocular pressure and glaucoma progression: results from the Early Manifest Glaucoma Trial. *Arch Ophthalmol*. 2002;120:1268-1279.

6   Fechtner RD, Realini T. Fixed combinations of topical glaucoma medications. *Curr Opin Ophthalmol*. 2004;15:132-135.

7   Woodward DF, Chen J. Fixed-combination and emerging glaucoma therapies. *Expert Opin Emerg Drugs*. 2007;12:313-327.

8   Kass MA, Heuer DK, Higginbotham EJ, et al. The Ocular Hypertension Treatment Study: a randomized trial determines that topical ocular hypotensive medication delays or prevents the onset of primary open-angle glaucoma. *Arch Ophthalmol*. 2002;120:701-713.

9   Weinreb RN, Friedman DS, Fechtner RD, et al. Risk assessment in the management of patients with ocular hypertension. *Am J Ophthalmol*. 2004;138:458-467.

10 Stewart WC, Stewart JA, Nassar QJ, et al. Cost-effectiveness of treating ocular hypertension. *Ophthalmology*. 2008;115:94-98.

11 Hitchings RA. A practical approach to the management of normal tension glaucoma. In: Grehn F, Stamper R, eds. *Essentials in Ophthalmology: Glaucoma.* Berlin, Germany: Springer-Verlag; 2004.

12 Khouri AS, Lama PJ, Fechtner RD. Beta blockers. In: Netland P, ed. *Glaucoma Medical Therapy: Principles and Management (Ophthalmology monographs 13).* 2nd edition. Oxford, UK: Oxford University Press; 2008:55-78.

13 Higginbotham EJ, Allen RC. Carbonic anhydrase inhibitors. In: Netland P, ed. *Glaucoma Medical Therapy: Principles and Management (Ophthalmology monographs 13).* 2nd edition. Oxford, UK: Oxford University Press; 2008:123-138.

14 Gabelt BT, Kaufman PL. Cholinergic drugs. In: Netland P, ed. *Glaucoma Medical Therapy: Principles and Management (Ophthalmology monographs 13).* 2nd edition. Oxford, UK: Oxford University Press; 2008:103-122.

15 Hejkal TW, Camras CB. Prostaglandin analogs. In: Netland P, ed. *Glaucoma Medical Therapy: Principles and Management (Ophthalmology monographs 13).* 2nd edition. Oxford, UK: Oxford University Press; 2008:33-53.

16 Flammer J, Haefliger IO, Orgül S, Resink T. Vascular dysregulation: a principal risk factor for glaucomatous damage? *J Glaucoma.* 1999;8:212-219.

17 Quaranta L, Gandolfo F, Turano R, et al. Effects of topical hypotensive drugs on circadian IOP, blood pressure, and calculated diastolic ocular perfusion pressure in patients with glaucoma. *Invest Ophthalmol Vis Sci.* 2006;47:2917-2923.

18 Bloch S, Rosenthal AR, Friedman L, et al. Patient compliance in glaucoma. *Br J Ophthalmol.* 1977;61:531-534.

19 MacKean JM, Elkington AR. Compliance with treatment of patients with chronic open-angle glaucoma. *Br J Ophthalmol.* 1983;67:46-49.

20 Kholdebarin R, Campbell RJ, Jin YP, et al. Multicenter study of compliance and drop administration in glaucoma. *Can J Ophthalmol.* 2008;43:454-461.

21 Olthoff CM, Schouten JS, van de Borne BW, et al. Noncompliance with ocular hypotensive treatment in patients with glaucoma or ocular hypertension an evidence-based review. *Ophthalmology.* 2005;112:953-961.

22 Granström PA. Glaucoma patients not compliant with their drug therapy: clinical and behavioural aspects. *Br J Ophthalmol.* 1982;66:464-470.

23 Baudouin C. Detrimental effect of preservatives in eyedrops: implications for the treatment of glaucoma. *Acta Ophthalmol.* 2008;86:716-726.

24 Pisella PJ, Pouliquen P, Baudouin C. Prevalence of ocular symptoms and signs with preserved and preservative free glaucoma medication. *Br J Ophthalmol.* 2002;86:418-423.

25 Rahman MQ, Tejwani D, Wilson JA, et al. Microbial contamination of preservative free eye drops in multiple application containers. *Br J Ophthalmol.* 2006;90:139-141.

26 Rouland JF, Berdeaux G, Lafuma A. The economic burden of glaucoma and ocular hypertension: implications for patient management: a review. *Drugs Aging.* 2005;22:315-321.

27 Rylander NR, Vold SD. Cost analysis of glaucoma medications. *Am J Ophthalmol.* 2008;145:106-113.